Fitness athlete, entrepreneur and social media entertainer Zac Perna has established a global presence in the world of fitness. Zac graduated from the University of Melbourne with a Bachelor of Commerce and immediately started his online fitness business and social media career amassing a following in the millions. Known for his comedic style and a desire to inspire and teach others, Zac has transformed tens of thousands of physiques and lives to date. He also owns a pyjama brand with his brother and lives in Melbourne, Australia.

# GOOD INFLUENCE

## Zac Perna

HarperCollins*Publishers*

**HarperCollins*Publishers***
Australia • Brazil • Canada • France • Germany • Holland • India
Italy • Japan • Mexico • New Zealand • Poland • Spain • Sweden
Switzerland • United Kingdom • United States of America

HarperCollins acknowledges the Traditional Custodians
of the land upon which we live and work, and pays respect
to Elders past and present.

First published on Gadigal Country in Australia in 2023
by HarperCollins*Publishers* Australia Pty Limited
ABN 36 009 913 517
harpercollins.com.au

A catalogue record for this book is available from the National Library of Australia

ISBN 978 1 4607 6467 1 (paperback)
ISBN 978 1 4607 1655 7 (ebook)
ISBN 978 1 4607 3654 8 (audiobook)

Cover design by Michelle Zaiter, HarperCollins Design Studio
Cover photograph by Jake O'Donnell
Typeset in Baskerville by Kirby Jones

To everyone in pursuit of the life they deserve, I hope these pages help you in some way on your journey to finding it.

# Contents

**Author's note:** this book includes general health and motivational advice but it's important you consider your individual circumstances and where necessary consult a qualified health professional before starting any new fitness, diet or resilience (ice bath!) program.

# Introduction

Hi, I'm Zac. We're about to have a conversation about how you can make a better life for yourself. It's going to be interesting, informative and funny, and it just might give you everything you need right now. Sadly, it will be quite one-sided in that I won't actually hear your responses, but just pretend like you're talking to that friend who never lets you get a word in. In any case, we'll get to know each other a lot more closely over the following pages, but first I'd like to take a moment to personally welcome you to the mental ramblings I'm so fortunate to call a book.

Let's cut the shit. You're probably asking yourself, why on Earth should I listen to this guy? The short answer is that you don't have to. A sexier answer, that's better for selling books, would be that I hold the blueprint for going from a scared, overweight and broke kid to becoming a confident and happy millionaire walking around in his dream body. But that answer may sound a bit corny and reek of unrealistic arrogance. A more heartfelt answer, that happens to be true, is that you should listen to me because I wrote this book for you. I wrote this book for the average person wanting to improve their health, for the experienced gym-goer seeking new perspectives, for those with ambition who want more out of life and for those who feel stuck in their situation – like I once did.

I don't regret anything that I've done in my life, because every event has led me to the very moment I'm in right now. With that said, it's my goal to extract the lessons I've learned, the mistakes I've made and the insights I've found along the way to set you on the path towards your goals and condense the process as much as possible. It shouldn't take you 10 years to change your life. You don't need to make the same mistakes I did to get in your best shape. You can be on your way to living your best life as quickly as you can finish the words on the pages to come. I am *excited* for you!

I wish I could tell you that I always had my life in order, but the truth is that I had my shit together as much as any holiday-maker in Bali drinking water straight from the tap. I was scared and lived passively as a result, letting life just happen to me. So what changed, you might ask? How did I suddenly take hold of my destiny with both hands and steer it into the life that I always wanted? Well, I am so glad you asked because it all started with a trip to Birmingham, England, and the birth of the Nando's Geezer.

## The Nando's Geezer

It's been a while since I've gone by the name of 'The Nando's Geezer'. It wasn't a name I gave myself, yet it's a name I graciously earned: it was thrust upon me by a random homeless man on the streets of Birmingham when I was in my early 20s. Finding myself on the other side of the world at that time in my life was completely my own doing, and became part of a lesson in strategy and work ethic that would stick with me for a long time. The seed that grew into this lesson was accidentally planted many years before, in 2016, by a man named Robbie Frame.

When I was signed by the supplement company EHPlabs in 2016, the dream was to have the honour of being flown to the biggest fitness event in the world: the Olympia in Las Vegas. I saw EHPlab's other big athletes getting to travel to the USA and stand alongside the biggest names in the industry. In my mind, if you were selected to go there, you had officially made it.

My mate Robbie was a big athlete for EHPlabs in Australia at the time, and he'd had the privilege of representing the company at the Olympia Expo previously. I asked him what it would take for me to be selected to go there. How many followers would I need? How could I prove myself worthy? His answer was an elegantly wrapped present filled with a box of common sense. 'Who knows? I asked them if I could go if I just paid my own way.'

What?! You can do that? You can just be a responsible adult and make your own way in the world without relying on someone else?

It sounds like absolute common sense, yet it isn't so common in today's world of entitlement and elevated self-worth. Very few people want to take charge of their lives; people want to be *selected*. Being important enough to be flown across the world is an ego stroke large enough to spike anyone's dopamine. But the simple fact is, no one's going to baby you and chase after you to make sure you achieve your goals. If you want something, you'd better be able to back yourself and be responsible for your own journey.

When I thought about it, I didn't need the ego boost: I wanted the opportunity. Just like Robbie.

I never made it to the Olympia expo, because EHP didn't attend for a few years. But I took Robbie's advice the first chance I got. When my clothing sponsor, Gymshark, announced that they would be holding their largest pop-up event in their hometown of Birmingham, I saw the chance.

They didn't invite any Australian athletes, because the cost of flying over a few Aussies would be exorbitant and unjustifiable. So I asked my contact if they would *allow* me to attend the event, alongside the other athletes, provided I paid my way. I was willing to cover flights, accommodation, food and even the hotel minibar (not that I would use the hotel minibar – no way I'm paying $11 for a chocolate bar). I didn't care what it would cost me to go, because the opportunity to be there was an investment worth every cent.

They agreed immediately and were even kind enough to cover my accommodation. I was genuinely shocked. I flew myself to the biggest event of my life, where I could greatly expand my network and improve my credibility as an 'influencer' and everyone just assumed I was important enough to be flown overseas with Gymshark. Not a single person asked me if I'd had to pay for my flights.

My trip to Birmingham was a huge success and one of the best decisions of my life. I made connections and friendships with the internal team and other athletes. It felt surreal just to hang out with these people that I'd looked up to for many years. To have one day had these athletes on pedestals and the next day be organising a casual workout as mates was unreal.

It's interesting to note that some of my best friendships have started at events like the one that Gymshark hosted. Although we come from all over the world, it often feels like meeting alternate versions of myself, who share the same interests, passions, problems and ambitions.

In any case, during that UK trip I filmed a bunch of things that boosted my socials and paved the way for future content creation. Shortly after, I would actually be flown to other pop-up events by various organisations – despite my continued willingness to pay my own way.

All in all, it was a great trip. I have many memories of the event, of the people I met and, unfortunately, of seeing a lot of homeless people. I would walk the streets of Birmingham every morning for my daily cardio routine, my gut filled with mixed feelings. Blended up in there was the worry that I was about to get the shit kicked out of me by some shady-looking individuals in hoodies, a daily desire for Nando's, and a sense of empathy in the purest form for the many homeless people out on the streets.

I combined two of these feelings into a video idea: I would buy a heap of food and give it out to the homeless. I'd seen this done before, though I was aware that it always seemed disingenuous when people give away food because it's being filmed. People are quick to comment that it's 'wrong', implying that if the content creator really wanted to help they wouldn't film anything and instead would just perform an altruistic gesture of feeding the homeless with nothing in return.

However, the world doesn't work like that. It's debatable whether true altruism can even exist if you gain anything by performing a positive act. If I give something to one homeless man, I feel better that I have positively affected someone's life. They gain a meal; I gain some positive feelings of warmth, and validation that I might be a good person. If I gave out twenty meals, I could feed twenty people in need, feel good about myself twenty times over *and* make a feel-good video for others to watch and experience joy when each person received their free meal.

I wrestled with the idea and concluded that it was the right thing to do. So one morning on my walk I asked a particular homeless man: if he could have any meal of his choice, what would it be?

Being homeless obviously doesn't give you the luxury of dreaming about food the way that most people do; he clearly hadn't spent too much time thinking about that question. Eventually he responded with 'any hot meal'. I continued to probe and he told me that hot chicken would be ideal. 'Like Nando's?' I asked. 'Yes,' he confirmed.

The next day I went to Nando's and bought hundreds of dollars' worth of meals: wraps, pitas, hot chicken, chips, drinks and sides. I walked along the Main Street and started handing it out to people in need, starting with my anonymous friend. I approached him with a, 'Hey mate! Do you remember me?'

'Ohhh right, you're the Nando's Geezer!' he said ('geezer' being informal British slang to describe a man).

Holding back a laugh at my new nickname, I confirmed the title and handed him a bunch of hot chicken and chips.

I'm not going to lie, the appreciation was something I'll

never forget and I'm so glad I was able to capture it on video (after asking the man's permission to film).

I continued on my way until I ran out of Nando's. I didn't think I'd get a more memorable response than the first man, but when I was down to my last wrap I decided to give it away to another geezer that I spotted sitting down. I approached him from my high horse and said, so helpfully, 'Here you go mate, here's some Nando's for you.'

Instead of a look of praise and gratitude, I was met with sheer bewilderment. He looked at me, confused, and said, 'But why?'

In that moment my eyes widened as I took in my surroundings. My brain felt like Bradley Cooper in *Limitless*, after his first dose of NZT-48. It took me half a second to realise that this man wasn't homeless but was actually a busker taking a short break from his musical performance. Fuck. I responded 'Ahh just ordered too much mate, thought you might want it. Cheers.'

I handed over the wrap and walked, as fast as possible, away from the luckiest busker in Birmingham.

My trip to Birmingham was proof that I didn't need to wait until I was deemed worthy or important. No one can afford to wait until someone else values them enough to build their dream for them.

This realisation wasn't a bad thing at all. It felt like a gift, similar to a nice peri-peri chicken wrap enclosed in thin, tightly wrapped paper. I *could* achieve things from my physical fitness, go places, be seen and make shit happen, and the choice to do so was entirely *mine*. I didn't have to wait for anyone else to take me places, nor did I have to wait for the right moment to make a move. I had concrete proof that, if I wanted to get out there and succeed, I could. A Nando's Geezer can make his own way.

So I did.

## Learn from me so you don't have to figure it out

Apart from being one of my favourite stories, becoming the Nando's Geezer was crucial to determining the intersection of my business ethic, commitment to health and fitness and my desire to help people and have it inspire millions across social media. I want to inspire you to stop waiting for the life that you want.

The structure of this book replicates the three key pillars of my brand: mental fitness, physical fitness and social media. While I encourage you to read the three parts chronologically, technically you can start in whichever order you please, as the sections all intersect and influence one another. Without further ado, here are the three parts:

**Part 1.** My transformative experience of 'mental fitness' where I learned to sustain good habits for life by building the mental foundations for happiness, success and consistency. I even dive into some philosophy here, so don't skip this – you're in for a treat.

**Part 2.** Now that you have the foundation of living your best life, here's all my tips, tricks and knowledge about physical health: from diets to exercise, I'll share how to change your life.

**Part 3.** Stepping into the wild world of social media and how I achieved financial success through multiple avenues.

I should also mention that woven throughout all of the above are stories of craziness, a strong dose of humour and an openness I've never shared with anyone before. So consider this your own personal (and hilarious) road map to becoming a lean and happy good influence in your own life. Let's begin.

# Mental Fitness

# 1
# Welcome to my brain

Mastering physical fitness is easy. Everyone *knows* what they should do to get in shape. If they don't, they just need to read over part two of this book and then they'll have a pretty decent idea.

If it's so easy, why isn't everyone out there living their best life in their best shape? Why do people struggle with adherence, motivation and consistency? It's definitely not due to a lack of information, because we all know that eating a dozen donuts probably isn't good. Why do we still experience so much difficulty? Because physical fitness is maintained in the mind. You need to focus on building the correct mental habits of self-awareness and other healthy practices as a foundation to your physical health.

Enter mental fitness. Getting mentally fit took a decade of making the same mistakes, neglecting my mental health and wondering why sustained happiness was always so hard. This change didn't happen overnight. I had to work for it through hours of dedicated practice, including reading, self-reflection and meditation under every full moon with a hand full of crystals. I'm kidding about that last bit; we'll keep it fairly straightforward when it comes to what to do. Point being, it took me a very long time.

Ideally I would like to help you fast track the entire process of building a healthy level of mental fitness. And believe me, some of the stories in this section are absolutely mental. Some of these pages reflect on important lessons of the mind that eventually laid the foundation for building my dream body, and others are helpful, weird or, hopefully, just simply interesting.

I hope that these stories can give you something to think about, make you laugh, directly or indirectly improve the quality of your life, and help you open yourself up to sheer possibility. We're about to explore the foundations that are vital to staying consistent, getting the most out of yourself and enjoying the process. So grab a towel … for your brain I guess? (I don't know. Don't judge me. I'm too deep in this analogy to back down now.)

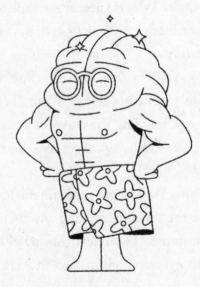

# 2

# What playing the euphonium taught me about adulthood

At my high school they had a program that allowed the new students in Year 7 to choose any instrument and receive free lessons for six months. This was music to my ears. I played guitar throughout primary school and to think I could learn another instrument for free was nearly as exciting as going to a new school. Without hesitating, I signed up.

I didn't care what instrument I'd learn, in fact musical instruments didn't even matter. I just wanted to dive head-first into everything the school had to offer. I'd come from a small primary school and all of a sudden I was part of this giant ecosystem filled with wonder and opportunity.

In my first week I signed up for the trumpet. Every Wednesday I'd have trumpet lessons for 30 minutes and then take my trumpet home with me for more practice. Sadly, my skills didn't match my enthusiasm and my teacher actually told me maybe my mouth wasn't suited to this wind instrument. Instead, he suggested I blow into something else … and my lessons were never the same again. His recommendation of the euphonium made it much better! The wider mouthpiece was easier to play than the tiny trumpet mouthpiece, which left me straining my pursed lips. Suddenly, I was a euphonium player!

If you don't know what a euphonium is, just picture a tuba (its cousin). I would take this on and off the bus with me and I didn't care in the slightest, because I got to play the euphonium for free and learn something new and cool (not actually very cool). I practised daily and, after six months, my teachers asked if I wanted to perform in front of an audience at the school's music show. I replied with a fervent yes.

So I practised even more. You probably know how the story goes: kid defies social norms, kid learns instrument, kid practises hard, kid performs, everyone loves kid, kid goes on to become child prodigy and shock the world with his talent. Well, I got the first couple! Only mine went more along the lines of: kid learns instrument, kid practises hard, kid annoys the living shit out of his parents, kid continues practising, parents want to stab pencils in their ears. Kid performs. Then, nothing.

I stopped playing the euphonium shortly after. Why? Because I had experienced it already and it was slightly boring now and there were so many other opportunities to be taken by the horns. So (while still in my first year of high school) I auditioned for a role in the school play. It was Shakespeare's *A Midsummer Night's Dream* and I was cast as one of the lead roles: Nick Bottom. I wasn't really a drama kid and the idea of auditioning was terrifying. But I did it.

I challenged myself with extracurricular activities and academic achievement. I won the Chinese prize out of all of the students in the year level and won an award for general academic excellence. I took pride in my schoolwork and never wanted to get below 95 per cent in any subject. I had my few friends; I made friends with anyone but I was far from one of the 'cool kids'. The cool kids played sport, I played large instruments that hurt people's ears. The cool kids ignored the teachers in class, I wanted to impress the teachers with my work. You get the point.

In fact, just a quick story: at our school one of the things Year 7s had to do was study a famous person's life (someone notable for a remarkable achievement) and then become that person for a night while the parents walked around and asked the students questions, which the student would answer in character. There were a lot of sports stars that night, musicians and legends in the room, and then there was me … wrapped in orange sheets, wearing a bald cap and glasses, posing as His Holiness the Dalai Lama. I looked like a complete psycho, but I didn't care! I was fascinated by Buddhism and thought it would be fun and interesting to be the Dalai Lama, (which it was).

I didn't know it back then, but in my first year of high school I was demonstrating my most powerful character trait. It took me 10 years to harness that strength again. It's a quirk of my personality: I saw the fun in everything, the opportunity in life to try new things, to not care what people thought and instead explore what I could do to reach my full potential. I remember thinking that I could do *anything* and I was so fricken excited about what my future would hold. The world was a huge place and I was ready to dive right in.

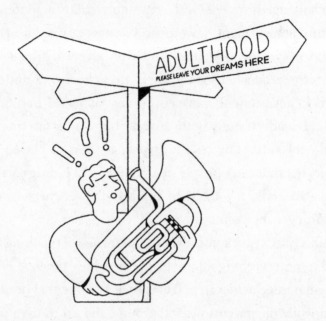

I'd love to see what would've happened if I maintained that mentality. But sadly, I did not. I lost it. I lost what made me *me*. All of my quirks were slowly dampened and silenced by the social pressure to fit in and be liked. So, after Year 9, puberty kicked in and all of a sudden it was important to be cool. (Side note: I still focused on academics. I never let that one go, as I had subconsciously attached a part of my identity to being 'the kid that gets good marks'.) Anyway, my priorities slowly shifted as I tried to become well liked. I wasn't disliked by anyone's standards, but I wanted to be *really* liked. Liked by the girls and popular around the guys – you know, pretty much the same mentality most kids my age had.

In hindsight, this wasn't my fault. Humans have evolutionarily adapted to want to belong to a group and feel a sense of acceptance. This is biologically ingrained in us. Our ancestors survived so long ago because they *were* accepted into groups and not left to fend for themselves. Sadly we cannot ask the descendants of the latter group for their opinion because … well, they don't exist. Poor loners.

I didn't realise at the time, but my longing to be well liked slowly suppressed the idiosyncrasies that made me the happy-go-lucky teenager I once was. For those wondering, I was in fact successful in my pursuit of social status. I made it to the popular group and navigated my way through high school relatively unscathed. Maybe if I never succumbed to social pressure, I would've had a far different experience. Kids could've made my high-school life hell on Earth. I'll never know. But I have seen that whatever you practise can snowball, for better or worse.

I focused primarily on academics and buried the other sides of me. I was accepted into the country's number one university as a result and studied commerce. University was different to high school. It was actually the opposite, now that I think about it. I arrived at university with that same need to be liked. Only I cared so much about what other people thought of me that I wouldn't speak to anyone out of fear of being disliked or embarrassed. I became shy and reserved. I kept to myself and went to uni only when I had to. The idea of capitalising on the uni's outstanding extracurricular program was daunting. So instead of throwing myself in at the deep end and signing myself up for every activity or club I could, I crawled back into my shell and let the feelings of anxiety take over.

University was my first real experience with anxiety. It hit me every time I got in my car to drive to campus. I felt like I was dumb and insignificant. I felt like the world was a huge place that could swallow me up any minute if I put myself out there. Opportunity turned into a stressor and I avoided being on campus (apart from classes) at all costs. It brings to mind the only quote I remember from *Coach Carter* for some reason: 'Our deepest fear is not that we are inadequate. Our deepest fear is that we are powerful beyond measure.' My own potential frightened me because I felt like I no longer had the courage to pursue it. Acknowledging what I *could* achieve would mean coming to terms with the fact that I had to step out in to the world and take risks once again.

The gym was my refuge and a place where I felt comfortable, so I used it as a crutch to get through uni. I couldn't make friends because talking about future plans would give me instant anxiety, considering I didn't know mine. Studying on campus made me feel like I didn't belong, so I would get out of there as quickly as I could to avoid another bout of inadequacy. I finished uni in the end, but it was not an enjoyable experience. Thankfully I was working on something else in the background.

At that point, I was posting religiously on social media and trying to grow my following on YouTube and Instagram. I had around 100,000 followers when I finished university, and I gave myself one year after graduating to try and make something happen. In fact, that timeframe was entirely arbitrary. If I needed two years to make it work I probably would've given it two years. A lot of people will give themselves 12 months to achieve a goal, but for what reason? Is your goal only worth 12 months?!

On the bright side, my social media presence was the best it had been. But my problems weren't over. I was still crippled by a fear of ambition and I refused to acknowledge it.

My parents are the most supportive people. They were constantly encouraging me to pursue bigger and better things (probably because they knew the kid that I was). I'll never forget one conversation I had with my mum in the car. We were driving to the snow one winter and I was telling her about the online coaching programs I had started writing for people for a few hundred bucks a week. I didn't have a business set up yet, so I was just doing what made sense to me. Mum suggested I start thinking about turning it into a proper business. 'Imagine,' she said, 'if you had your own app and platform to put your clients on! You could create a community on there and take it global! You'd crush it, how good would that be?'

And do you know what I said to these words of encouragement? I turned to her calmly and said, 'Please Mum, can we stop talking about this? Because it's freaking me out.' I wasn't excited by the idea, I was scared of acknowledging my own potential.

My family continued to support me and didn't push too hard. They knew I was ambitious deep down and just needed time to find that ambition. It's funny looking back now and seeing that I took my mum's idea only a few years later and turned it into a million-dollar business. Oh, how I wish I could go back to that day and say, calmly, 'Mum, you're a fucken legend.'

I think most people can benefit from harnessing that childlike sense of wonder that once made them true to themselves. The playful version of ourselves that brings fun and joy to life that far too often gets lost in the things that don't truly matter. I lost that part of myself for a while and only in the last few years have I got it back. I lost it because I let the bullshit get to me in high school. I let people tell me that the world is big and scary and you shouldn't try things because what if you fail?

Well let me tell you what happens if you fail. You play the metaphorical euphonium. You pivot, you see what else there is, you explore every opportunity you can and you get fucking excited about what you can do! Because if you're reading this then you have the opportunity to do something great, whatever it is. Even if it's playing the most annoying instrument known to man until your household wishes you just stuck with the damn trumpet.

---

# 3

# Count your wins and give 'em these ones

Frankston station was the end of the line from Southern Cross Station in Melbourne. The train would depart the city and embark on its journey to pick up some of the most damaged and troubled individuals and take them to their final destination, where they could plague the streets freely and without care. It was a land where scoundrels were free to roam, which bad lads would call home: a true paradise for any young thug, bully, mugger or hoodie. The kind of place that would make me run, not walk, to my car and lock the doors as soon as I shut them. Have I set the scene dramatically enough?

In Frankston's defence, I can definitely think of worse places in Melbourne. The focus here is on Frankston for two reasons. Firstly, it's where I chose to work every day in my early 20s, and secondly, it's where I started off my 'dream job' in the supplement industry. Actually, before we delve into what happened during my time working in Frankston, let's rewind to even earlier than that to my first full-time job.

I had just graduated from high school with an ATAR score of 95.9 and an acceptance into my first pick of university. This was a moment I had worked my ass off over six years for, yet the excitement was short-lived. Like most other kids, I was now faced with the difficult question of, 'What do I want to do with my life?' I also had no money.

So, with that fantastic start, I began my first full-time job at a pharmacy, buying time to enjoy my gap year before starting uni and facing the question I tried so hard to avoid.

In the beginning, I loved it. I was able to talk to random old people about protein powders and would jump at the sight of anyone pacing up and down the sports nutrition aisle, hoping I could persuade them into talking to me about my only hobby. The chemist saw my passion for bodybuilding and gave me the responsibility of the entire sports nutrition aisle. They soon noticed the care I took in my work and gave me the responsibility of the confectionary aisle. Pretty opposing positions, now that I look back on it, but at the time I pretended like this was the most important task ever and made sure we hit record-breaking sales of lollies due to my constant stacking and facing of the shelves.

After a year of work, I figured out what I enjoyed (talking about protein) and what I didn't enjoy (justifying to old ladies why I had to look in their handbags). Theft was actually quite prevalent in the pharmacy, but you'd be surprised at how much old ladies don't give a fuck about your problems as long as you don't look in their bags. I wonder what they even had in there that was worth screaming at me over.

Anyway, I left the job and applied for something more suited to my ambitions. I avoided the strange zombies surrounding me and handed in my résumé at Australian Sports Nutrition (ASN) in Frankston. I wanted to be as perked up as possible, so before walking in I chugged my pre-workout to let the caffeine elevate my dopamine and bring out Chatty Zac. Instead, the caffeine stimulated my adrenals more than the increased dopamine and brought out Shaking and Terrified Zac. I spoke to the manager, and I swear to God he stared so far into my soul it left the building and jumped on the next train back home. Somehow he saw something in this panicked kid and I got the job.

I was living my dream, talking to people daily about their fitness goals and how best I could serve them through supplements and nutritional advice. I became a supplement fanatic and knew what ingredients made a great pre-workout and what flavours burned sales. I was finally able to spend half of my week doing something I enjoyed and learning more about the industry. During the other half of the week I went to uni to study business. I must admit, it was quite strange talking to the Frankston residents. A moment I won't ever forget is being told by one of them how meth actually makes a great fat burner (not my recommendation).

We had a lot of shady characters walk into the supplement store. Maybe they were lost, or perhaps they just wanted someone to talk at (there isn't a lot of two-way dialogue when you're talking with someone on meth). Anyway, this one particular encounter always stuck with me.

A wrinkled, dishevelled-looking bearded man came into the shop once. He might've been anywhere between the ages of 45 and 70. It was impossible to tell. He asked me about protein and creatine to support his muscle growth. I asked him if there were any other supplements he was taking. Boy, I'm glad I did. It turns out this old dude's doctor had him loaded up on steroids to promote weight gain. This 50kg dude was juiced to the gills with pharmaceutical-grade testosterone.

In complete shock after hearing his 'stack' (this is what bodybuilders call someone's supplement regimen), I asked him what kind of training he was doing. Was he going to the gym or just home workouts? He responded in a slurred Aussie accent, 'I do it all at home with me watering can … I just fill it up and then give 'em these ones –' he moved his arm in a clockwise, circular motion '– then I take some out and give 'em *these* ones,' he said, moving his arm counterclockwise this time.

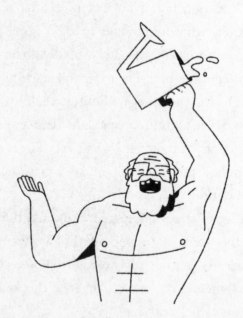

This demonstration continued for an enjoyable five minutes as I wrapped my head around the fact that this guy was slamming gear while watering his garden for exercise.

I tried to tell him that he'd be better buying some weights or joining a gym, and that his watering can probably wouldn't cut it, but he seemed fairly content that I was the one who didn't understand the anabolic effects of 'giving 'em these ones'. He hobbled out of the shop and I remained perplexed at the conversation I had just had. I couldn't get the image out of my head of this guy watering his garden harder than I trained.

Tricky characters aside, I did enjoy working there. I would constantly look at all of the new products on the shelf and imagine what it would be like to have my own brand there. If I thought working at a supplement store was a dream, this was really *the* dream. Little did I know that only a few years later I would in fact have my own product on there and in hundreds of other stores too. The product is called Pride and I made it in conjunction with EHPlabs (my supplement sponsor).

I had been working with EHPlabs since I started in fitness. They were the goal brand and I aspired to be a part of the company from the beginning. After a few years of working with them, the owner, Iz, flew down from Sydney with a team of videographers to make a short documentary piece on me as an athlete. It's quite rare for the CEO of a company to fly down to get involved with such a small part of the business, but that's what Iz was like. He would constantly oversee decisions and ensure that the brand (his baby) would continue to succeed and flourish. He and I also got along really well, so I think he just came down to hang out for a bit.

Coming from my background of selling supplements and his background creating supplements, we began talking about new products and ideas, one being the ideal pre-workout. I feel like it was on a whim he said, 'We should make one together.'

I couldn't really take him seriously because he just so casually said what had always been my absolute dream, but I entertained it nonetheless.

We spoke over sushi and he would turn my input of feelings into the output of ingredients in milligrams. After a few minutes we had a formula on a napkin for the collaborative product Pride.

Just under a year later I was flying to Utah with Iz and his family to see where the product would be made and to try the very first samples. I *still* couldn't believe it was actually happening, but as usual I entertained the possibility and ran with it. The product we created was unreal and exceeded my expectations.

When it finally landed on the shelf and online I think it all finally hit me. My name on a tub of pre-workout was now a reality ... only my awe and excitement slowly fizzled as I became concerned with the next goal: how can we enable as many people as possible to experience this?

I had new goals and a new measure of success. Don't get me wrong, I was excited, but just like my 'dream job' at ASN, I took it and moved on to the next goal. It was like my baseline of pride (in the literal sense) and happiness had shifted upwards with the more things that I did. The journey and the idea of doing big things was what stoked my fire and made me hungry for more, whereas achieving any one particular thing was not as exciting.

I think most people can relate to this feeling of disillusionment when achieving something does not generate the high that you thought it would. It highlights the role of dopamine in the search for a desired outcome. To me, this shows the difference between happiness and contentment. The feeling of excitement and happiness is what I would get instantly when thinking about the new opportunities I was working towards. I would get this dopamine hit whenever I was pursuing the goal or when I achieved a small win from it (such as going overseas to formulate the product). The only downside is the dismissible fact that this feeling is fleeting. Contentment on the other hand is more of a long-lasting feeling produced by serotonin and, in my opinion, gratitude. It isn't transient and it lasts much longer. It's unaffected by ambition and leaves you feeling warm inside, like there's no place you'd rather be.

I'll illustrate with an example from my own experience.

When I got out of school I wanted to work at the chemist to talk about protein and get discounted supplements that went out of stock. I was so happy about this. But I wanted to talk more about supplements and even get free products on occasion. So I got the job at ASN and was so happy about this. Then I jumped at the chance to have my very own product and get paid for doing so, and you can bet that I was *so* happy about this. But like every preceding event that gave me happiness in the short term, it wasn't enough to keep me content. I was constantly beset by the next goal, the next objective that would *truly* make me happy. Having my name on Pride wouldn't make me happy, what would make me happy is if it became the nation's bestselling pre-workout.

But in fact nothing would ever take me to true happiness and I was constantly chasing the never-ending rainbow.

In a way I think it's a good thing that the human mind has a bias towards seeking more. It's probably what caused our rapid evolution as a species. Imagine if we sat back and thought, 'Jeez we've reached the pinnacle of technology with these bone-spears guys. Let's just chill.' We wouldn't be here now – if we were, I'd be communicating this entire book to you via grunts and interpretive dance.

Some people will argue that it's this constant dissatisfaction with life that propels them further. I do see it! If you're always hungry, you'll always eat. But on the other hand, I think such a mindset creates a life of discontentment and a feeling of the grass always being greener. Like anything, there are two sides to a coin and one must delicately manage the balance of it to keep the coin spinning. This is something I've had to work on personally and I have done so through goal setting and gratitude practices.

Goal setting will increase my ambition and desire for more. In this mindset, growth is the vision and I want to reach the upper limits of my potential, and then keep pushing. Gratitude practice, on the other hand, involves sitting back and reflecting on where I am now and how far I've come. One simple gratitude practice can immediately change my state of mind and give me a new perspective on life.

Try it now. Take note of three things that you're grateful for and try to truly feel the emotional weight of it. You'll notice your mood shift.

It's for this reason that the practice of gratitude has become an integral part of my day. I do it so that I don't take things for granted or let my ambition drive me without any balance from the other side of the coin. Something as simple as writing down a few things every day that are going well in my life or something I'm truly thankful for goes a long way. Even a bigger picture gratitude practice done less frequently works. Practising these together I am able to recognise my aspirations for more while also being proud of what I've managed to do. These two contrasting mindsets have enabled me to enjoy both happiness and contentment at the same time. I can then reframe my mindset from, 'This is no longer good enough. I want more,' to 'I'm grateful for this opportunity and proud of what I've done. Let's see what else we can do,' without feeling disappointment or loss in the process.

I've learned that if I can't be truly grateful for what I have, then it doesn't matter *what* it is that I want, because acquiring that will never make me truly content – whether it's a university degree, a dream job or more money. I also learned that you can get absolutely fucking jacked if you lift a watering can every now and then while giving 'em these ones … apparently.

# 4

# Using stoicism to become mentally unbreakable

I never knew how much money could be made from selling iPhones on my social media. To make thousands of dollars, all I had to do was post an Instagram story informing people that I was selling a new iPhone for just under market value and they would PayPal me $800 to purchase. I had already built up enough trust in my audience for them to take my word for it, so my followers knew a good deal when they saw one! I sold around 13 iPhones in half an hour and made over $10,000.

There were a couple of downsides. Firstly, it was not actually me behind my Instagram account selling phones. I had no idea it was happening (I was actually at Woolworths doing some grocery shopping at the time). And secondly, the iPhones being sold didn't actually exist: the hacker was making bank from my trusted audience. I remember putting my shopping bags in the car and getting a few texts from mates asking if I was actually selling my phone. I thought someone had pranked me somehow until I couldn't log in to my Instagram. Great. I had just managed to grow my Instagram to a point of monetisation and it was taken away from me in the time I decided which bananas I'd like to buy.

Thankfully, I knew a guy who was able to log the 'genius' hacker out and grant me access once again. I changed my password and told every buyer to cancel their PayPal payment, along with directions to their nearest Apple store to have another 'genius' sell them an iPhone.

For a whole 30 minutes I was jobless … and it was utterly terrifying.

My brain has always jumped to conclusions and overthought things. As a kid, a typical train of thought when my parents went out for dinner would be, 'I wonder what they're eating … Wow it's almost 8.30 … I hope they haven't been in a car accident … They definitely got in a car accident … Holy shit, I'm an orphan.'

I'm not kidding, that's where my mind sent me. It wasn't too different over a decade later, when my mind spiralled out of control in a Woolworths car park and I felt like I had lost everything. My chest tightened, I felt the blood rush to my face, my breaths became shallow and my throat swelled as I felt the fear consume me. I had no ability to see another perspective on this potential lifestyle change. I couldn't see the flip side: in my mind it was all bad.

My brother was different. Now for those of you who aren't familiar with me, my brother Joel is my best friend. He'll crop up a lot in this book, so pay attention. Now, Joel didn't have the same attitude towards life. He outgrew the feelings of loss aversion and took on a more optimistic outlook in the face of adversity.

Wait, let's go back a step. *Joel* was actually the one who devised the theory that if Mum and Dad went out by themselves they were 100 per cent destined for a car crash, with over 98 per cent confidence and a p-value less than .05.

However, as I said, my older brother outgrew this. If he was presented with a challenge or hardship, he would take it on the chin. He would take a measured approach and understand that it's never the end of the world, it might just be a little bit shit. While I was worried about my social media being hacked, Joel was working 10-hour days building house frames. If you don't know what that entails, imagine getting up hours before the sun, lifting obscenely heavy objects in the rain, losing feeling in your hands as you carry yet another wall across a job site and getting home after dark. He had his own business and worked six or seven days a week just like this for a very long time, until he couldn't do it anymore. He knew that something had to change, but he didn't know how.

If that were me at that time in my life, I don't think I would've had the balls to even *think* of doing something else. We find comfort in the known, even when it's crushing us. But Joel saw options in the unknown, and instead of thinking, 'It's been seven years, what else could I do?' he thought, 'It's been seven years. Fuck doing this for another 30.'

Most people can relate to the former thought. They use past

commitments to dictate what they should do in the future. It's a human bias that affects our rational decision-making abilities; we hate feeling like we've done 'all this work for nothing' and the longer the duration of time committed, the harder it is to break the habit. It's like watching a movie you aren't enjoying after the first 30 minutes bored you to tears, but you've already committed 30 minutes of your life so you may as well spend another 90 minutes miserable. When you put it this way, it seems quite illogical and that's because it is.

It has a name: the sunk cost fallacy. People struggle to get past this, and as a result can get stuck in the rut of doing things that cause pain and misery just because they've already committed time to doing so.

Long story short, Joel made the decision to pursue something better. It took a while for him to figure out what to do exactly, but it had to be something that sparked excitement. He settled on the clothing industry. After one conversation, we *both* decided to make pyjamas. Two Aussie lads in their mid-20s with zero experience in the rag trade and a goal to make the best pyjamas in the country.

We had no idea how to do this, but ever since we had the idea to create Slouch Potato, Joel became a new person. He worked for a few more months to save money and then quit his job to figure out a way to make pyjamas with his brother. If it wasn't for him I definitely would not have jumped out of my pool, but seeing his excitement and enthusiasm was inspiring then and it still is today.

It's like for some reason my default emotion was set to pessimistic. Thankfully the brain is remarkably adaptive and you *can* change your mindset. I just had to have enough self-awareness to recognise my thought patterns and whether they were helpful or not. Joel's brain was set to optimistic. He figured that despite his current circumstances and past experiences, today is a new day to do what you love and no one else is going to change your life for you.

When he did quit, he said something to me that really resonated. He said that even though he had spent seven years doing something he no longer wanted to do, he had zero regrets. Instead, he just started reeling off lessons from his challenging experiences, which any rational person would assume to now be a waste of time. He said it taught him resilience and proved to himself that he could work harder than others. It instilled in him a sense of independence and confidence knowing he could throw himself into something so difficult and emerge successful. It taught him how to manage staff, how to motivate people and, in that stressful time doing something that brought him so much pain, it taught him to value the things that truly mattered.

Not a waste of time at all, but it depends on how you look at the situation.

Joel is my inspiration. We teach each other things every day. I taught him how to construct an Excel spreadsheet and he teaches me how to be a better person. Pretty much even, if you ask me! In all seriousness, working alongside him really instilled a sense of optimism that I try to carry with me every day when faced with challenges or difficulties. Understanding that each outcome has both negatives and positives is crucial. Drawing out the lessons from the hard times prevented me feeling like I was helpless and instead granted me control.

Stoic philosophers live by the principle that no event is either good or bad, it's just what you make of it. They will dispute the idea of any event being bad. If your car gets stolen, great, you can now ride a bike to work and improve your fitness. Stoics draw out the lessons and opportunities in life. Reading about this philosophy and practising it daily has singlehandedly changed my life, because I know that I am not a product of circumstance; rather I can choose how to approach a given situation.

It's not easy. There are times when I still feel like the world is caving in around me if something goes wrong, only now I can recognise the thought and immediately counter it. I think, 'WWJD (what would Joel do)?', or 'What would the ancient stoics do?' I try to see it from a new perspective. Without sounding like a preachy self-help guru who sits around all day smelling his own farts, if you practise framing your problems with this mindset, you will feel more in control of your life and not chained to feelings of helplessness.

The mindset has two components. Firstly, it's about detachment. The next time something seemingly bad happens, pause. Take a breath. Understand that something neutral has happened and you've chosen to *perceive* it as bad. Then try to detach yourself from your perception and explore other alternatives. Find a positive in the event and know that you can always take away something from it, even if it is just a lesson. Epictetus (the famous stoic teacher) said, 'It is not events that disturb people, it is their judgements concerning them.' The second component is much easier to do: control the controllable and accept what you can't.

I find this mindset gives me a great deal of relief in difficult situations. My mind always seeks to fix things and control outcomes. When I can't control the outcome (yet still try to), it gives me immediate feelings of stress and restlessness. So instead, I separate what I can control from what I can't. Whatever is out of my control I just try to accept.

The idea that we are the only ones who ascribe meaning to events that befall us can be either daunting or empowering. When something bad happens, it's easy to blame external factors, overgeneralise, search for permanence in the situation or blame yourself. These are belief patterns that lead to helplessness and depressed thoughts. What I find fascinating, however, is the role that mindset has in transforming one's state in spite of the circumstances. Take an average guy or girl, for example. If he or she loses their job, they could immediately resort to negative beliefs about themselves and the world, such as, 'I'm not capable, I always ruin things, I'm not worthy' or 'I'll never get a job again', and they would perceive the event as disastrous.

The stoic, on the other hand, would perceive job loss as neutral and control their perspective of the event. They might choose to perceive it in a positive light instead of a negative one. The stoic might see the opportunity in the challenge of finding a new job, the chance to try something else, the chance to learn from their experience and at least walk away having grown or experienced something that will make them a better person.

Joel and I would often joke about the famous stoic emperor Marcus Aurelius getting told his mother had passed, and responding with a delayed '... This is good.' Dark jokes aside, the simple lesson is the underlying idea that you are in complete control of your state of mind and how you perceive the world.

Stoicism is like playing Jedi mind tricks to grow as a person, thrive and be happy, instead of resorting to a default negative mode every time something perceivably 'bad' happens.

So, back when my Instagram was hacked and I was locked out of the platform I'd spent years building, my job was taken away from me in an instant and I almost let it crush me. If that were to happen to me now, I would be in a much better position to reframe the situation. I would recognise my immediate stress response and then be able to see it as a *perception* of the event, not the event itself. I would then figure out what I could control (finding someone to retrieve my account), what I couldn't control (the outcome) and be ready to accept the situation. In my acceptance, I could then look for the opportunity the event presented, just like Joel did when he was at his lowest. Then, as a very worst-case scenario, I would realise that if all else fails, I could always just quit everything and make a living selling iPhones.

# 5
# Get bloody cold

Falls Creek is a ski resort located between Victoria and New South Wales in Australia. It is a cold yet picturesque location, home to snowy mountains and a lake that's often either fully or partially frozen over during the winter months. In 2021, a few intrigued skiers and snowboarders on the Towers Chairlift might have turned around to see three snowboarders ride past the lift line, off the track towards the half-frozen lake, take off their boards, snow gear and thermals, slowly walk into the lake wearing only undies and slip into the freezing-cold blue depths. Those idiots happened to be me, my brother Joel and my cousin Luke.

Joel and I had been practising cold exposure for a while and wanted to test it in the most raw and primal conditions. Luke hadn't had a cold shower in his life but was up for the challenge. Despite the water being just above zero degrees, we slipped in and calmed our minds and heart rate until the water felt like simply nothing.

I remember stepping out and feeling the sun's heat like it was a scorching day in peak summer. It was amazing what Joel's and my bodies had become used to in just months of consistent cold exposure. Luke, on the other hand, waddled in waist deep and saw his heart rate climb to 200bpm before he painfully waddled back out to avoid a potential cardiac arrest (the video is on YouTube for those interested).

Practising cold exposure is a non-negotiable in my daily routine. I have extreme adventure athlete and all-round interesting person Wim Hof to thank for that.

Wim Hof was the first person I had heard of practising extreme cold exposure. He held records for the longest underwater frozen lake swim and seemed to have mastered his body and the elements. He once completed a marathon in the desert without any water. From afar, he seemed like the least relatable human on the planet and a true genetic outlier, but I was too intrigued by his story not to read his book.

In *The Wim Hof Method* he talks about how cold exposure and breathing practices were game-changing in controlling his mind and body.[1] It's an amazing read for those interested! Before reading his book I had never had a cold shower for longer than 10 seconds in my life, but following his protocol I 'warmed up' to 30-second showers, increasing in 10–30 second increments every day. After a week I was having two-minute showers relatively pain free and I noticed a benefit. I actually filmed a YouTube video documenting the process, and you can see after my first cold shower I had an immediate smile on my face.

I didn't know it at the time, but I was increasing levels of dopamine and adrenaline in my brain, causing a rush of feel-good neurochemicals. I also didn't know it at the time, but after posting that video over three million people would see me in the shower.

I kept up my cold showers. I made it part of my routine to step from my warm bed into a cold shower. It didn't matter if it was summer or winter, I would get it done. Not to be a hero or anything, but more for myself: I was addicted to the feel-good chemicals that would come after the cold. My mood would be better and I would be more energetic and ready for the day. I also enjoyed the feeling of mental resilience. I wasn't going to be a comfortable weakling wrapped up in his warm blankets; I wanted to tackle something uncomfortable every day for my own sense of strength.

After a while, however, the body becomes adapted to the cold routine and you require even colder temperatures to elicit the same feel-good response. So Joel and I bought an ice bath and I would take the plunge into an eight-degree tub every day. I would avoid it only when I was getting sick, as it seemed to make any early symptoms of sickness turn into something much more serious.

Interestingly, Wim's other method, of breathing with deliberate hyperventilation and breath holding, is believed to alleviate sickness and help the body fight it off, potentially due to acute increases in adrenaline from the breathing activity itself. It's truly an addictive habit that I think holds plenty of upsides, provided you don't have an underlying heart condition and do it responsibly.

The benefits of consistent cold exposure can be broken down into physical and mental. Among the many proven physical benefits, my favourite would have to be the increase in dopamine.

Cold exposure can elevate the body's baseline level of dopamine for hours.[2] So instead of temporarily spiking dopamine like a recreational drug, resulting in a steep crash and feeling like a piece of shit, the increased dopamine is more of an upward shift of the entire curve, not just a huge peak. For me, this meant an immediate improvement in motivation and mood (hence, why I like to do it in the mornings). Other interesting benefits can be an increase in brown fat stores (more metabolically active fat tissue) and improved circulation in the body.

The mental benefit for me is the resilience I mentioned earlier. I wanted to be constantly happy with seeking discomfort, because no one succeeds by remaining in their comfort zone! Ironic from someone who sells pyjamas and preaches the importance of being comfortable, but I think we need a bit of both, right?

I challenge you to jump in a cold shower tomorrow morning. If the weather is cold and you're warm in bed beforehand, even better. It's best if you really, really don't want to do it, then force yourself to do it. Control yourself and have the discipline to stay in there for your goal time. If you can't do that just one time, you have bigger issues. But once you do, you'll notice how freeing it is to draw on the discipline and mental resilience you didn't know that you had. It's a pretty cool feeling (pun intended)!

I actually contacted Wim after my video went viral. I told him that I was going to do a 'day in the life' video based on his routine. Ideally, I would have travelled to the Netherlands to spend some time with the legend himself, but it was peak Covid so a Zoom call had to suffice. I told him I just needed 10–15 minutes of his time and we ended up chatting for an hour about many subjects: his beliefs, goals and vision, and answers to any questions I had on his routine. He even performed one of his rap songs for me. It was awesome to chat and he was quite hilarious.

After spending months wondering, I had to ask him if he still felt the cold. I wasn't sure if he would be used to it after so many years. Would cold even feel cold? Would it feel nice? I just had to know if it got easier – I knew what to expect with ice baths, but it really hurt. His answer made me laugh out loud as he emphatically said, in his Dutch accent, 'Of course it's painful. IT'S BLOODY COLD.'

I guess the discomfort never leaves and it's not so much about removing the discomfort but more about being comfortable with its presence and improving your ability to deal with it. His energy and vision for the world was highly contagious and grateful for his time, I thanked him for paving the way and promised to continue spreading the message.

In the beginning, a cold shower will feel extremely uncomfortable and an ice bath will feel like you actually might die. I've coached dozens of people in an ice bath and noticed that every time a client gets in for the first time, they all have one thing in common. They feel incapable of sitting in there and certain that something horrific will happen unless they get out. 90 per cent of them look me dead in the eyes and say, 'I can't do this' before jumping out like a cat that accidentally fell in the pool.

This belief in their inability is what interested me, because of course they *can* do it, but all of them were certain it was impossible. I would coach them through their next session and try to change their perception of the event.

*Breathe deeply and slowly. Focus on the sensations. What are they? How do your calves feel? What about your upper legs? Your arms? Lean into the feeling and realise what it truly is. Is it a pain on your skin? A tingle? Can you do this for another three seconds? Of course you can, because you're doing it right now and you're fine.*

This mostly gets people through their first minute, and it allows them to focus on the present without catastrophising. Usually the body signals danger and the brain will urge you to get out so that you don't die. But if you condition your mind to stay with it and be present, you'll realise that nothing bad will actually happen in the two or three minutes of sitting there.

Then you get out of the tub (or shower) and you are flooded with dopamine and adrenaline. You feel mentally capable because you exceeded your expectations for yourself. You also feel mentally resilient because you controlled your mind enough to not give in to primal urges. After a few weeks of practice, you realise that it's not going to kill you and it is just bloody cold. So you deal with it. And in 'dealing with it' you are able to improve your physical health and grow in the process.

**DO THIS:** start with cold showers. Aim for 30 seconds every day and slowly increase the time under the cold until you can handle three minutes (which is the sweet spot for optimum benefits). Practise calming your mind and overcoming the urge to get out. Then graduate to even colder waters, like an ice bath or the ocean.

# 6

# Why you need to be scared

Growing up, my brother and I would constantly scare each other. I couldn't turn the lights out without knowing there was a good chance that Joel would be waiting in the dark, and he couldn't turn a corner in the house without the fear I'd be behind it ready to jump out at him. After we watched *The Nun,* I printed out a life-sized picture of her face and stuck it to his window. We'd both go to extreme lengths to get a scare; there is still nothing quite as sadistically satisfying as scaring a sibling. But this time Joel's face was like permanent fear staring me right in the soul.

It was still quite funny.

He sat opposite me on a flimsy seat in what felt like a tiny metal room with wings, 13,000 feet in the air. He had begun mentally preparing himself to jump and begin his plummet back down to Earth at terminal velocity (around 200km per hour).

I write this as if I wasn't also absolutely freaking out. I was scared, but my brain didn't let me believe that I was jumping out of a plane. The view from the window looked so similar to a regular flight, and just like every other time I've caught a plane, the height isn't real. It no longer feels like a dangerous height and instead becomes just a nice view. But when I saw Joel immediately get ripped out of the plane, the realisation kicked in.

Approaching the open door, I barely had time to think. The instructor strapped to my back told me what to do without giving me a chance to question it. 'Okay stand up, hold that, hold this, ready – OUT.' I had a few seconds to realise what I had signed up for, but he didn't even let me think, he just told me to stand up and grab the bar. Before I knew it, I was flying.

Skydiving was hands down the scariest and most awesome thing I've ever done in my life. When my feet hit the ground I felt like I could do anything. Adrenaline aside, there is a seriously good feeling doing something that scares you. I've spoken to Joel about it since and he told me that ever since he started *seeking* fear, things got better. Not in the sense of extreme sports and dangerous activities, but small things on a daily basis. Public speaking is terrifying, even for me who's *technically* used to talking to millions. Difficult conversations are scary, as we know we might not have the words and ability to remain composed. Trying something new and risking failure is horrifying.

We fear judgment from others and judgement from ourselves, because if we fail, then what does that say about our identity? We feel like a loser, so it's better to avoid the whole scenario altogether, right? Well, only if you want to remain where you are.

Joel began searching for things that scared him because he knew that it made him a better person. I was signing myself up for an acting course, and Joel said he would do it too, purely for the reason that it found it absolutely terrifying, but he imagined a version of himself that wasn't scared – that's what lured him to want to do it.

It reminds me of what I did in high school, for no explicable reason at the time. I signed myself up to play guitar and sing in front of my entire year level. For someone who doesn't really sing, that is a proposition only conjured up in the most stressful of nightmares. I didn't really explain to anyone else why I did it and I'm not sure if I fully realised it back then, but in retrospect, the reason is obvious.

Girls.

I'm kidding, I did it because *not* doing it would feel like backing down from an opportunity at gaining a life experience. It scared me, so my gut reaction was to say no and find an excuse. For whatever reason, at that time, I despised that part of me that was so scared of life, and so I did it. Interestingly, the worst thing that happened that day was a couple of sniggering kids when I didn't hit that high Jack Johnson note. I gained some respect from my peers for putting myself out there, and most importantly I felt better about myself for doing it. I was one of the few people who was willing to face it head on.

Confronting a fear is not just 'pushing' your comfort zone, but expanding it. Your comfort zone goes from a small circle to a huge one, encompassing things that you never thought you could do. I never thought I could jump out of a plane. In fact I'd pretty much ruled it out, despite wanting to. When I did it, I proved to myself that, if I can do that, I can do anything else that terrifies me: I can be the type of person who constantly expands my comfort zone. If I was getting ready to film a daunting video in public, I would say to myself, 'You've jumped out of a plane, this is nothing.'

It doesn't have to be that extreme. I will do the same mental gymnastics every time I face another fear. If I were to give a huge talk, I might remind myself that I did the last one just fine and therefore I can succeed again. This mentality has enabled both my brother and I to accomplish things we didn't think we could. It kind of feels like a superpower. In reality, what's taking place is an expansion of our own references of what we think we're capable of.

The more empowering references you have to look back on and base your capabilities off, the more you will accomplish in general. Acknowledging the silver lining in any fear-inducing situation allowed me to feel like I was on a path to constant growth. So I learned that fear is good. Fear acts as a stimulus for me to become a better person. Obviously not all fear is equal, and there's not much to gain by cutting my leg and jumping into shark-infested waters, but I think that goes without saying.

There's obviously a connection between fear and danger, but it's up to the individual to discern which activity is dangerous and should be avoided and which activity is in fact harmless and should be confronted head on. Again, the risk and reward always has to be weighed. Skydiving, for example, has a risk of death of 1 in 100,000. Statistically speaking, you're actually twice as likely to die playing American football than you are skydiving out of a plane. You're almost 50 times more likely to die choking on food. But of course you accept the odds and justify the risk of choking for the reward of not starving to death.

That's a stupid example and I should've just said that I justified the risks of skydiving with the experience it would give me.

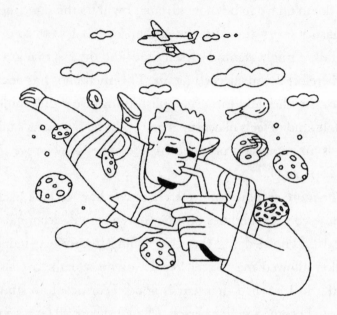

My relationship with fear taught me to pick up the camera and talk even when I was suffering from anxiety, which enabled me to make my first YouTube video. I can't tell you how scared I was filming. I had the goal of making videos to help people and bring fitness into people's lives, but the barrier was a crippling fear of talking to the camera and filming. It never came naturally and my earliest videos looked like dash-cam footage of a deer in headlights. But, slowly slowly, I faced my fear every single week, until it no longer felt scary.

I've filmed myself in public for hours interacting with people. Recently, for a dare, I filmed myself hosting a public fitness class in the middle of the shopping centre. (The joke was that I would be hosting a fitness class with no one attending, yet still screaming, 'Come on people, feel the burn.' Horrific and cringeworthy, but I did it and felt great afterwards.) If I never faced my fears as a 21-year-old kid with a camera, I never would've built the career and life I have today. And after my new experience with fear, I have become an impenetrable fortress immune to fear.

Okay, maybe whenever it's too quiet in the house I'll still raise my voice and call out to the darkness, 'JOEL, YOU BETTER NOT BE FUCKING WITH ME ... I KNOW YOU'RE THERE.'

# 7

# The daily habit that changed my life

It was 2019 and my sponsor Gymshark was in the middle of hosting pop-up stores in huge locations in major cities, and for some reason they wanted me at the one happening in Manchester in the UK. So, without any delay, I accepted the 24 hours of travel and began what turned out to be another surreal experience.

Many other athletes and I around the world would head to the one location, meet fans of Gymshark, host seminars and mini events, and just have fun. It was always such an awesome vibe. I walked into the athlete room on the first morning and saw my good mate Matt (mattdoesfitness) talking to this muscular, intimidating-looking bloke with arms bigger than my head. This was Ross Edgley, the man who had just swum around Great Britain, and it wasn't until I heard the cheeriness in his voice that he seemed less intimidating and soon became someone I wanted to talk to. So I stepped into the conversation to see if I could keep up with the general gist.

Matt was in awe of how someone could swim around Great Britain, for 157 days straight. To which Ross replied enthusiastically, 'Yes, but it's also the same with your food challenges ... It's so impressive to me how someone can have the mental resilience to consume *that* much food!' Yes, Ross just compared his death-defying test of mental resilience, where he was eating 15,000 calories per day to perform the swim, to a 10,000-calorie food challenge. Matt nodded in apparent agreement, smirking because we were both thinking that you absolutely cannot compare the world's longest swim to eating a few donuts and burgers on YouTube.

This was just Ross, though. He was unbelievably positive and would seek to pump people up and bring positive energy to the room. So, back home in Australia, when he sent me a copy of his book documenting the swim, I was all for it. I wasn't reading a lot at the time, however. I read as a kid and loved it, but the habit probably died with the numerous torturous books forced upon me in high school. For that, I blame my teachers, mice and men and also twelve angry men. So I hadn't finished a book willingly for a few years, but I was prepared to try and pick the habit up again.

I sat down one morning and began Ross's book, *The Art of Resilience*. He spoke about his journey at sea intermingled with his philosophical beliefs on stoicism, which, at that point, I had never heard of. I obviously now employ stoicism to help my mindset, if you skipped the chapter head back to page 32 now.

I was so intrigued. I would read every morning as part of my morning routine. Even 20 minutes of reading would have me feeling absolutely pumped. I gained perspective and it forced me to internalise certain principles of mental resilience. I was hooked. I finished his book in a couple of weeks and went down the rabbit hole. I traced stoicism back to the millennium-old books of Epictetus, Marcus Aurelius and Seneca. I then branched out into the work of Cal Newport and James Clear, on productivity, and various other books on business, psychology, happiness and inspiring life stories.

It felt like I had just found a superpower to be able to live inside someone's head for a week and absorb their thoughts. I read every morning and evening. There was no way I would skip out on learning as much as I could and enhancing my perspective of the world. My morning books were the ones to influence my daily thinking (so business and psychology), whilst the evening books were more general interest (science, biographies or fiction). I read on average a book per week for the next year and noticed my mindset completely shift. I even forced my brother to adopt the same habit, and he was the furthest thing from a recreational reader. Edgley's book might have been the first book Joel read voluntarily, but once he developed the habit, he was the same as me, and we would share books, our thoughts on those books and what we personally would take away from the work.

Reading is the one habit that I've stuck to for years and I attribute quite a lot of success to it, even if it's not success in the monetary sense but success in being a better person. It took me out of the bubble that I was living in and gave me perspective and ideas from hundreds of other people. I constantly tell people that they should try reading as part of their routine. My advice would be to do it first thing in the morning, when the world isn't demanding anything of you yet. Just get up 20 minutes earlier, sit in bed if you like, and give yourself over to reading a book. Your day will improve, your mood will improve and you'll see things positively – and that will open you up to opportunities and ways to better yourself. I don't think you'll get the same self-improvement from reading *The Hobbit* as you would from books on psychology, but if reading something completely fictional starts your habit then go for it.

Plenty of people tell me that they would like to read, but they just can't finish a book. To which I say, start with *any* book that you like. Hopefully you're starting with my book. (This is weird. I'm writing about reading for you to read, even though you probably are the only person that doesn't need this advice.) In any case, I'm baffled when people tell me they can't justify the time to read a book; the author has spent far more time writing it and pouring their ideas into it than it takes to read. So I'm of the opinion that reading someone's book is the least I can do.

As many habits do, this simple positive habit bred even more positive habits, like meditation, journalling and now writing. I just needed a catalyst to kickstart it into gear. I've read over a hundred books since that day in Manchester. So if you're not an avid reader, then I urge you to finish this book and move on to another. If you are an avid reader, I'm now nervous. You've read plenty of books and now you're reading mine. That's utterly terrifying. I hope you like it at least. Do you like it? Don't answer that. Now I'm forgetting things. Fuck. How do I end a chapter again? Surely not like this.

# 8

# The optimal morning routine

Fewer things are less practical than an influencer giving advice on how the average person should structure their day. Influencers: technically unemployed, somehow have more than 24 hours in a day with fewer responsibilities than a typical pet owner. So it's not all that inspiring to squeeze in a hot yoga, sauna, hair appointment, workout and plant-watering session, all before 12pm.

I personally consider myself an entrepreneur and content creator as opposed to an influencer, but most people choose not to distinguish one from the other if the person in question has a social media following. It's for this reason that I've always been very hesitant creating content for the average person about setting up ideal routines. No one can adopt every piece of advice and what's helped me may not help the next person. However, one caveat I will always mention is that it is futile to aim for perfection but to aim for an improvement in your daily routine. Improving my morning routine changed my life. It improved my mood, I had better days, I felt happier and more motivated and I experienced less anxiety.

I mentioned earlier that my anxiety would often be brought about by ambitious thinking (goal setting, future plans, big ideas – you know, the fun ones). Yet when I focused on improving what I do in the morning, the anxiety subsided and I felt capable and in control. This is why I am compelled to dedicate time to spreading the message to others online. Hearing other people's stories of life improvement would be fuel to continue helping others with this.

The first person I saw a positive change in after addressing their routine was my brother. As I have mentioned elsewhere, I urged him to begin reading. From someone who was a terrible reader, now Joel's favourite time of the day is his morning read in bed. It sets him up for the day and makes him feel like he has some time to himself.

Instead of telling you what to do, I'm going to tell you what I do (and have done for years) that has improved my life. My morning routine typically consists of these things:

## Avoid my phone

I realised early on that there was one task that had accidentally become part of my morning routine, for the worse.

Checking my phone was instinctive in the morning. I'd wake up, tired-eyed and with brain half-asleep, and reach for my phone, scrolling through updates I missed overnight. Instead of catching up on anything useful, I'd just expose my mind to everyone else's highlights and be left feeling useless in bed.

My brain would still be in half-dream/half-awake mode and anything I would see on my phone would cause me to overthink and believe irrational things that I'd carry through my day. So that was the first thing that had to go from my routine. I have a rule to set my phone on 'do not disturb' and I CANNOT open it unless I have finished the last step of my morning routine.

## Read

I replaced my morning social media scroll with caffeinated reading. They say you shouldn't ingest caffeine too quickly, but I personally can't ingest it quickly enough. I love my time waking up, sipping some coffee and reading in silence for 10–30 minutes. As I mentioned in chapter 7, I'll read a non-fiction book in the morning. Something to get my brain working and thinking positive thoughts. I believe the brain is quite malleable in the morning and whatever you 'feed it' will set the tone for the day. In other words – at the risk of sounding like I am holding energy crystals – positivity begets positivity. Once my reading is done, my mind will have had enough time to wake up and come back to Earth. Then, iPad in hand, I'll begin my next phase.

## Day planning

For those fortunate enough to have flexibility in time and structure in their workday, this is huge. I dedicate a few minutes to jotting down the things I would like to get done in that day, in order of priority, whether that's work, fitness, life admin or anything else. Even just taking the time to figure out what's important to me that day is very powerful in adding purpose and fulfilment to my day.

I also ensure I do this before someone else tells me in an email or message what I must do. For example, if I wake up and decide on my own terms that I'm going to prioritise working on my fitness clients in the morning, I don't want anyone else to sway this – for example, if a boss, business partner or friend needs something done that isn't urgent. Unless it's essential I will stick to my plan and work other things around it (not the other way around). Obviously there will be things that I'll need to factor in and change; however it's important for me to not let anyone else run my day. Waking up and checking your phone does the opposite. It signals that you're responding to the demands of the world and reacting to stimuli.

I realised that people are always going to ask things of me. And while it may be my responsibility to complete them, it isn't my responsibility to complete them at the convenience of others and to the detriment of my own happiness.

## Cold shower

As outlined elsewhere, having a cold shower is my favourite way to add a small spike of adrenaline to the morning. It's painful, but it's the fastest legal way of adding some mental resilience and immediate wakefulness.

It's only after this step that I'll consider looking at my phone because my day has been (roughly) outlined. Most importantly, I'm awake and mentally alert.

I'll sometimes add additional activities to these steps, such as breathing exercises (Wim Hof method) or an actual workout, but it depends on my morning and how much time I have. A meditation has crept in there before, but I prefer to add that in my evenings to wind down and not draw out my morning routine to over an hour. These four simple steps take me around 40 minutes to complete, so I usually get up an hour earlier than I *need* to.

Joel did the same thing as a carpenter: he found that he had to get up at 4.30am just to get these steps done, and 3.30am if he wanted to train before work. Unbound by any additional responsibilities like raising a family or studying, he would just get to bed earlier when possible.

As I said, there's nothing more aggravating than a stranger who doesn't know your life telling you how you should structure your day, so I've refrained from giving too much advice here and instead just outlined what helped me. At the risk of contradicting myself, I encourage you to do two things that most people would agree aren't too much of a stretch. One: identify and remove where possible any toxic or negative habits that you may have accidentally incorporated into your routine. For me it was the morning social media scroll. I can't see a place for this no matter your circumstances. Two: find at least one thing that you can add to your morning routine to promote positivity in your life.

If you would like to add any of these steps to your day, I would suggest you start slow and work on building each one as a habit. Don't commit to 30 minutes of reading and a three-minute cold shower; just do five minutes reading and a 30-second cold shower. Once the habits are in place you can increase the duration of each one relatively easily. The old cliché of small steps leading to big outcomes rears its smug face in discussions like this.

Don't discount the effect that something as small as leaving your phone alone on the bedside table for 15 minutes can have. Try and improve your morning routine ever so slightly and see the greater impact unfold. Oh, it's also imperative that you include an hour-long goat yoga, half an hour of tarot card reading, two hours of positive affirmations and three hours of self-indulgent journalling about how amazing you are.

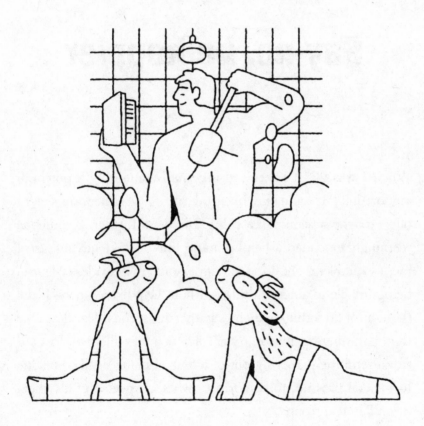

# 9

# Say no, be happier

When I was 20, if I received an email containing a potential 'opportunity' I would most likely take it, or at least hear the sender out – maybe schedule in a call to discuss it further. If someone seemingly extended a helping hand only to take advantage of me, I would let them do so out of personal insecurities or fear of being unable to achieve things without help from others. If the thought of attending a friend's gathering seemed less desirable than jamming my nuts into the stack of a lat pulldown, I would still attend the gathering out of a fear of being disliked or due to societal pressure to conform to what's expected of a typical 'friend' in the group.

Most of us grow out of young naivety, but I believe that my experience in social media accelerated this growth. Having any position of influence causes people to try and take advantage for their own personal gain, and as a result I was forced to say no to most people's requests. More 'friends' would message me out of the blue once I had something to offer and more people would continue to take from a relationship without giving anything in return. Hundreds of online hustlers would email me asking for money, disguised as a business enterprise, and in the end I either had to learn to say no or continue living to please other people. So 'no' became my favourite new word.

I also started to pay close attention to demands on my own time and see time as a form of currency. I would go into the grocery store to buy handfuls of groceries and when the register operator asked, 'Cash or card?' I'd simply respond with a dramatic pause followed by the word '… time' and confidently walk out of the store, bags in arms, leaving the operator perplexed.

In all seriousness though, let's compare the concepts. Imagine that a colleague or friend just randomly asked for $100. Depending on your generosity, financial position or attitude towards the person, you might say yes. They do nothing to repay the gesture, give no thanks and no good comes from it. The next week they ask for $150, and the pattern continues. Now at some point, any rational person can see the injustice in the situation and will eventually cease giving altogether for the sake of their own financial and mental health.

Money here is analogous to time, as both can be given, taken, invested and drained. People typically don't value their own time as much as their money. This causes others not to value your time either. For example, my journey into the fitness industry stemmed from my love of helping people change their lives through fitness and health. So when a friend (let's call him Steve) would ask for advice, I'd go above and beyond to help him. I'd spend hours writing meal plans and working with Steve's schedule, only for him to ignore the help, continue eating shit and message me months later asking for the same thing all over again. No matter how much I gave, it would never be enough. I know he didn't value my time because he never acted on my advice.

This was a harsh truth to realise. People will use a plethora of excuses to mask the fact that they don't value your time. If you let them continue to take advantage, it's proof that neither of you value your time. In the end, whenever Steve asked for a new diet, I invested no additional time and simply referred him back to the last meal plan. I also ensure I'm not 100 per cent reachable, at all times, to absolutely everyone. I have to set boundaries for myself and others. Don't get me wrong, I'm more than happy to give free advice or time to people, but with the condition that it's either appreciated, respected, acted upon or reciprocated. If not, people continue to take advantage until I'm left wondering why I'm so drained.

I had to learn how to say no to protect my own time, and to metaphorically say no to friendships, associations and false relationships to protect my wellbeing. This is surprisingly simple. You know which friend puts you in a better mood as soon as you see them, the one that leaves you feeling better than you were before, and you reciprocate happily. You also know which person leaves you feeling emotionally drained, zapped of all joy, motivation or happiness, and yet you may continue to call both of those people friends. At one point I realised that I don't actually need to feel drained and demotivated after every encounter with someone. So I started hanging out with the people who made me happy, the ones who made me a better person, and I stopped hanging out with the time wasters and happiness drainers.

I personally am always empathetic and want to see the good in everyone, so cutting ties with people or saying no is difficult for me. I feel like I have a moral and social obligation to say yes. It sounds kind of harsh but sometimes miserable people don't want to get better and simply want to bring others down to their level. The friends who gossip, talk about themselves, use, manipulate and leave a trail of havoc are the ones that need to be distanced.

Why? Because you are not responsible for other people's happiness, you are responsible for your own. Just like in an aeroplane when you're trying to ignore the robotic safety procedure, the oxygen mask rule somehow overpowers the noise cancellation of your headphones. You know, the one about placing your mask on yourself before trying to help others? Now I don't usually take everything said on planes as gospel (somehow a life jacket under my seat doesn't seem like very helpful information when plummeting to Earth), but I digress. The point remains that if you don't look after yourself first you are in no position to help anyone else.

For me, looking after myself meant saying no to toxic relationships and miserable people, and devoting more time to making the already meaningful relationships all the more meaningful. Respect your own time. Set boundaries. Know when to say no and don't neglect your own mental health in the pursuit of fixing someone else's.

# 10

# The crippling 'all or nothing' mindset

I was getting ready for my final Year 12 exam. The teacher instructed us to do a few practice exams to familiarise ourselves with the material, as these were all available online and dated back decades. I didn't end up doing a few. I did all 45 of them. It wasn't out of a fear of failing my exams, it was just my personality type, which leans more towards 'all or nothing'. I would throw myself completely into one thing and disregard any negative repercussions When I was at school, this was my work.

I didn't experience blowback from this tendency until I started getting heavily into the fitness world. I would train seven days per week for six months straight. I didn't go out with friends much because I didn't want to break my diet, and when I *did* go out, I would binge drink because I felt like the damage was done already and I might as well go 'all out'. I know many people can relate to this and some wear it as a badge of honour to hit the world hard with an 'all or nothing' mindset, as I once did. Usually, these are the ones who are yet to feel how brutal it can be when the world hits back.

After being in the fitness industry for a while, I continued to feed my obsessive personality, developed a subtle type of eating disorder, accumulated various anxieties and slowly approached a burnout phase in a physical and mental sense. I had seen countless fitness models abandon their social media platforms and disappear off the face of the Earth. Every now and then someone would say, 'Hey whatever happened to that shredded guy?' It was always a surprise to me. I couldn't understand how someone with *just* a social media following could go off the grid and retreat to a cabin in the woods away from technology or social interaction. But with any job comes certain pressures.

In the social media space, the pressures that you face are ones we were all taught never to care about: how you look and how popular you are. Social media influencers are primarily concerned with looks, particularly in the fitness space, because it is largely superficial in nature. The freakish bodies and the attractive people get the attention more often than not. Thankfully, there are very successful influencers that have been able to transcend the superficial layer of the industry through value-adding content that enriches the lives of others.

The pressure of popularity still remains, because if no one cares about them and they're losing relevance, followers and engagement, their job is at stake. If they're not popular they will generally make less money, unless they're quite savvy with their business (for example, one could thrive off monetising only a few hundred followers if done correctly, as opposed to many thousands).

For me, this pressure is inherent in day-to-day working life. I would say that it's the main disadvantage of the job. The desire to stay lean and in shape because your career depends on it is a very different motivation than because summer is around the corner. As is the desire to remain relevant and popular online due to it being your livelihood and not a hobby. Before I gave any thought to these things, I just continued to do more, take more work on and think that somehow these problems would dissipate. Only they didn't.

One day I just fell on the couch and quite literally threw my hands up. The thought of a cabin in the woods far from society sounded like bliss. That was my first experience with psychological burnout. Ignoring stressors and continuing to do more work didn't solve my problems, they just suppressed them until the problems all came out at once. Knowing I needed to change, I eliminated what I could and made my plate a little cleaner and more manageable, even if it was just temporarily. I needed time to relax, destress and take stock of my life to make sure I didn't just use the 'all or nothing' mindset of *doing more* to solve my problems. I realised that I could work my way through, but only to a point. I needed to incorporate designated times to relax instead of hoping things would change.

The same can be said about physical work in the gym. A lot of gym newbies fall in love with it and end up sacrificing everything for the gym. I did this for many years until I realised that it was damaging my gym–life balance. In fact, I shouldn't even use the word balance – my life *was* the gym.

Most people are familiar with the idea of work–life balance, because it's all-pervasive in society. Everyone can relate to being so caught up in the world of work that whatever is left of you is starved. And you have nothing to give to the people around you. The same thing applies in the gym – because of the transformative and obsessive nature of fitness in general. It's addictive, rewarding, comforting, fun and satisfying, and it changed my life. But just like a household painkiller, anything in excess is dangerous, even the good things. If you have 1000mg of paracetamol in one day, you might alleviate a headache, whereas 12,000mg will be lethal. In a similar manner, if you incorporate the gym and good eating habits into your lifestyle, you will improve almost all areas of your life. Whereas if all you do every single day is eat and train like a bodybuilder, you'll possibly be on your way to becoming miserable, selfish and alone.

I've seen plenty of bodybuilders who isolate themselves by never going out, never experiencing life outside of the gym and meal prep. In their minds, they are a hero, sacrificing luxuries and pleasures others enjoy so that they can endure pain to harden their minds and sharpen their bodies. In reality, they're only depriving themselves.

Don't get me wrong, I'm not against self-discipline. The world needs more of it. I'm talking about the extreme ends of the scale here. Imagine a spectrum going left to right depicting people's relationship with fitness. On the left lie the absolute sloths of the world. Those who have never so much as *read* the word discipline, let alone practised delayed gratification for a greater goal. On the right we have the aforementioned hardcore bodybuilders. Clearly the ideal would be somewhere in the

69

middle or perhaps a little over to the right. Those on the far right of the spectrum, who deny friends' social occasions and make the world about them and acknowledgement of their own pain and suffering, are just assholes.

I've seen fitness bring this out in people. It all starts from submitting to the 'all or nothing' mindset and judging others who do not. Have you ever seen a fitness enthusiast be utterly condescending when they talk to people who are happy to go out on a weekend and enjoy themselves? It's not very pleasant and screams douchebag. Thankfully I was never the condescending type, but I very much remember finding comfort in the fact that I would train seven days per week and wouldn't *need* other people. As long as I had the gym I was okay.

Now I can see how destructive this was. I wonder what would've happened if I'd injured myself so badly that the gym was no longer an option. If I had become so incapacitated that I couldn't rely on my meal prep and daily gym session to validate my identity, would I still not require friends or a social life for comfort?

It was only after the age of 24 that I put considerable thought and effort into adding more 'life' to the scale of my gym–life balance. I would catch up with friends even when it wasn't time for my dedicated 'cheat meal'. I would take a day off every few days and enjoy relaxing my body and resting my nervous system. Small changes helped me get more out of life and break the rigidity of a fitness-obsessed mindset.

Our bodies have an interesting way of dealing with environmental stressors. Once triggered, our bodies release hormones to deal with the stress (primarily adrenaline and cortisol). In the short term, this is usually beneficial and allows us to feel on-edge and alert. Then the parasympathetic nervous system kicks in and relaxes the response to bring us back to baseline. However, those with chronic stress do not return to their baseline as well. They experience more consistently elevated levels of adrenaline and cortisol. The effects of chronic stress range from anxiety and depression to high blood pressure and an increased risk of cardiovascular disease (not to mention cortisol's fat-storing proclivities).

We need rest. We are not robots that can continue delivering quality output, day in, day out, as long as we are given the right inputs.

And just because you can handle something for one day doesn't mean you can repeat it daily for years on end. Take a break. If you can see that you have an obsessive 'all or nothing' personality, be mindful of it and know that it's even more important for you to practise resting and giving yourself a break every now and then, whether that's from work, the gym or any other potential stressor.

I learned from experience that my mind and body need to be in a very specific state to continuously perform at a high standard. I can't work late into the night, get no sleep and do it all again the next day. My work will turn to shit if I don't get enough quality sleep and enjoy at least a couple of hours of relaxation before bed. So I deliberately shut down my work right before dinner. That way I *know* my work for that day is done. I can then reflect on the day and see how I managed my time and how I might need to manage my time differently tomorrow. I've learned that doing an extra few hours of work to accomplish a task will not be worth it in the long run and I'd much rather complete it in my designated working hours when I'm performing at my best.

Now obviously this advice is not applicable to everyone, and for some the luxury of relaxing at night remains a dream. The mum juggling working, putting children to bed and a baby waking up at 2am can't afford to walk out of her job and tell her kids to put themselves to bed because she needs some fucken shut eye. Some people have side hustles they're trying to grow, families to be responsible for and multiple jobs they need to get through. Some of these are short-term periods of GO that require one to put their head down and get through. It's like sprinting: you can do it for a while, but no one can sprint forever. You acknowledge that it's difficult but that it also mustn't last. Pencil in time to relax, socialise, treat yourself or just escape to a cabin in the woods if need be.

Just make sure it isn't *The Cabin in the Woods* cabin in the woods, otherwise you'll be dealing with bigger problems than burnout.

# 11

# A psychological battle of losing weight

I was standing backstage, covered in fake tan and demolishing Nutella-covered rice cakes. All I could think about was water. When you're about to step on stage at a bodybuilding competition, you want to get the leanest, driest look to your physique, and I was told water manipulation was key for this. (In natural competitions it doesn't really do much. It actually risks you looking worse – stringy and empty – for a 1 per cent chance of looking leaner. I shouldn't have cut water in hindsight, but the damage was done!)

In other words, I had just finished a six-month dieting phase and I was only concerned with the fact that I hadn't drunk any water in 16 hours. My body was telling me that if I didn't hydrate quickly, I was probably going to die. I suppressed the thought and stepped on stage when my name was called to perform the posing routine I had practised for many months prior.

Standing out there in my tiny blue budgie-smuggling posing trunks, I waited for my song to play so that I could begin the choreographed flexing and show off six years of training. A lot of hours in the gym had been leading up to this moment and I was ready. Only the music never started. The DJ looked at me, holding my USB stick like it was a piece of alien technology and mouthed the words, 'It won't play.' I felt like running over there and sticking the USB stick where it would fit (and likely then looking at *him* perplexed, wondering why it wouldn't play). But instead I responded with what felt like a yell: 'JUST PLAY ANYTHING.' Thankfully his seven brain cells obliged and he played a random song for me to continue my routine.

The nerves remained but I finished the routine, won my teenage division and then won the novice division in the ANB Men's Bodybuilding. Without sounding arrogant, I feel like I objectively deserved the win that day for combining muscular fullness with overall balance and also conditioning (low body fat). I was the leanest I'd ever been in my life. My triceps were feathered ('feathered' being visible muscular striations under the skin, not part of my progressive transformation into a bird) enough to make a kookaburra jealous. My quads were cut with anatomical lines I never even knew existed and my cheeks receded back into my skull, giving me the look of an emaciated rat.

And I still felt fat. This was when I learned that no matter how lean you are, in a quest to lose weight you will *never* be lean enough.

Dropping body fat is a lengthy process. We physically can't burn the 7.7 calories for 1g of fat than at the specific rate our bodies are programmed to lose it at. If you wanted to burn

1kg of body fat in a single day, you would have to burn energy equivalent to swimming for 18,000 metres. If you don't like swimming, you would have to walk 118,000 metres. And for the cheeky ones out there who may not like walking, well you could just have sex for 35 hours straight!

Now some of you reading this are wondering how someone can condense 35 hours of activity into 24 hours, and you'd be right: it's impossible. The rest of the guys are reading this wondering how someone could possibly exceed 35 seconds.

My original point being: fat loss is a lengthy process and can't be done in a day. It takes multiple days together to form weeks and months to even *notice* a change. This is partly due to you seeing yourself every day and creating a new reference point as to what you look like, and partly due to the nature of fat loss. This is why it's so important to not drive yourself crazy staring in the mirror every day, but to stick to the course of action and trust its process. You can't eat perfectly for one day and expect to be perfectly shredded the next, but after many more days combined you can. This is good in the sense that you can adopt a routine, create better lifestyle habits and over time be rewarded for your efforts. But the slow nature of fat loss is also dangerous due to the nature of incremental change.

Many people like using the frog and the water analogy to illustrate the danger of incremental change being imperceptible to the person experiencing it. The idea is that if you put a frog in boiling water, it would jump out as soon as it felt the heat, as opposed to incrementally heating the frog in the water to the point of boiling it to death. Firstly, why would you even boil a frog? Sounds like a very twisted experiment without a delicious outcome. Perhaps a lobster would be more fitting. Secondly, and much to my dismay, it simply isn't true. Being thrown in boiling water would be bad news for the frog, and many reptile and amphibian experts defend the frog's intelligence and report that it would actually get the fuck out of the water once it got too hot.

But let's pretend that the myth is true for a second, because it depicts fat loss perfectly. You burn fat at such a slow rate that over time you don't realise how lean you've become. In the early days that was me. I simply did not believe I'd lost so much weight. I believed that I just had to reach x level of body fat and *then* I would consider myself lean enough. It took me competing to get down to an unhealthily low body fat percentage to realise that I would never be entirely happy if my goal was to become as lean as possible. I would never be lean enough – I realised that this wasn't a physical problem so much as a mental one.

At the start of my diet I would grab a chunk of belly fat and pinch it. Probably a decent handful. I'd think, 'I have plenty of fat in here.' At the end of my diet I could still pinch some body fat on my lower stomach. Even though it would be the tiniest amount, I would still think to myself, 'I have plenty of fat in here.'

So how does one cure this mindset? You can't really. I think you just have to accept some level of body dysmorphia in order to beat it. For example, when I'm getting leaner, I acknowledge the fact that I *am* getting leaner, even though I am not 100 per cent satisfied with the level.

I try to separate my subjective opinion of my progress with the objective truth that I am losing body fat and the process is working. This is going to sound funny but, in my life, this means taking shirtless photos when I don't want to (I always feel unworthy of shirtless photos unless I am bone-shredded). I realised that if I take a photo when I think I'm 'not lean enough', in the future, I will look back at it and think, 'Wow I looked great there!'

It's like I live in a body that cannot communicate with itself and constantly changes its mind. One day it hates me, the next day it doesn't hate me and actually thinks that I'm great. It's like a crazy ex: they break up with you one day, only to come back months later *begging* for you to take them back because they didn't realise how good they had it … Admittedly that has never actually happened to me before and my exes probably moved on and settled happily with someone who doesn't say, 'Thanks, you too!' when the waiter says, 'Enjoy your meal.'

Like me, you might have to consciously apply this throughout regular day-to-day life, because once you begin your fat-loss journey you might start believing that it's not enough. Instead of chasing the rainbow, try to enjoy the process and over time be aware of the positive signs of progress. Notice how your clothes fit much better, how you feel much better and any other body changes. It's worth saying that these changes are not to be obsessed over but just something to be gently aware of.

So now that you're aware of the mental state needed in a dieting phase, you might be wondering what the best way to diet is? Well, keep reading – we'll get to diets soon enough. And note: this is where it gets more complicated than a DJ fumbling with a USB stick.

# 12

# The body's superpower

It's a strange thought that just five centuries ago, instead of worrying about burning fat or feeling great, our ancestors were gravely concerned about who in the village might in fact, be a witch. Hundreds of thousands of innocent women were tried for witchcraft, and even a few hundred men. Not a great time to be Harry Potter, or an HP fan – the franchise just isn't worth being burned to death over. One of the methods of trying a witch was 'waking', where a suspect would be kept awake for days on end by various means. Days of sleep deprivation would occur and ultimately end in a confession from the witch. The 'interrogators' would nod their heads in agreement upon hearing detailed admissions of flying around on broomsticks.

What was actually occurring was obviously not witchcraft but the hallucinatory effects and cognitive impairment caused by sleep deprivation. Later, many governments would utilise sleep deprivation as a method of torture and interrogation. I remember hearing an old story about a small group of people

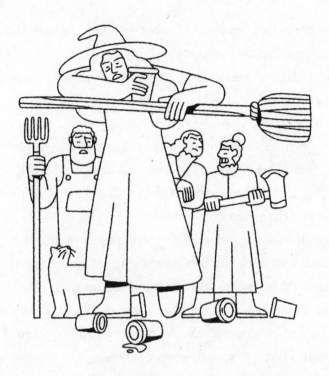

being locked in a room and deprived of both sleep and food, while other people watched their every move. And no, it wasn't a prison punishment or a twisted game designed by Jigsaw; it was actually a 2010 study by the University of Chicago to measure the effect of sleep deprivation on weight loss.[3]

Participants were placed in a 600-calorie deficit for two weeks while given 8.5 hours of sleep, and then 5.5 hours. The results found that both groups lost the same amount of weight, only the group that slept 5.5 hours lost half the amount of fat compared to the longer sleeping group and instead lost more lean body mass.

That study came as quite a shock. I'd spent years waking up early to get my cardio in, only to be left wondering if I was eating into my muscle mass in the process. Would I be better off just sleeping? Like millions of other people, I never prioritised sleep and it turns out my body did not like it.

You probably know what happens when you're overtired. Your focus suffers, you feel stressed, you make bad decisions, you seek out unhealthy food, you move less, your temper worsens, you get brain fog and you feel generally more miserable or less happy. Poor sleep is also a fast way to ensure an early grave, increasing the risk of cardiovascular disease, type 2 diabetes, cancers and depression.

Still, all those negatives didn't stop me from launching into stimulants and pursuing a constant state of wakefulness, never mind that I'd be constantly tired and anxious, and less able to cope with stressors. When I was in my early 20s, I thought an enduring sense of doom was the way my brain worked. I now know that if a single stressful event is feeling like the end of the world, I probably just need more sleep. Only in the last few years has sleep become a huge priority in my life, not only for its obvious mental benefits but for the aforementioned physiological benefits too.

In short, the body will simply function poorly in all aspects when deprived of sleep. So how can you improve your sleep? Through the two components of sleep quality and sleep quantity. Quantity is the simplest: it is generally known that adults need approximately 7–8 hours of sleep. Quality of sleep means ensuring you experience each stage of a sleep cycle. One cycle lasts around 90 minutes, and we cycle through them usually four to six times per night. Within each cycle, there are two phases of sleep: rapid eye movement (REM) and the other phase, which is creatively called non rapid eye movement (NREM). REM sleep contributes to improved cognitive function, memory formation, healthy testosterone levels and brain health, and what we'd consider 'feeling good'. NREM sleep contributes largely toward cell repair in the body and is when deep sleep occurs, which is needed for recovery and a healthy immune system.

During the first half of the night, we spend a longer time in NREM (deep) sleep. That is to say, if you get in bed at 2am, you are likely missing out on some important physiological benefits of deep sleep. Or maybe you can get to bed early, but you can't stay asleep for long and therefore experience a reduction in sleep.

Either way, there are no hacks or shortcuts to bypass low sleep quality. If you are sleeping poorly or not sleeping enough, something has to change. So how can we address sleep quality? Firstly, by controlling what can disrupt sleep and optimising what can aid it.

Around the time that I worked in retail, selling supplements, was the peak of my love affair with caffeine. Disclaimer: please do not try anything I am about to mention as it can be very dangerous and is *never* recommended. In fact, it's completely idiotic.

I would wake up in the morning with a double scoop of my caffeinated 'fat burner', equalling 300mg of caffeine. That's around five shots of espresso. I'd then head to work and be surrounded by samples, so I'd try another fat burner. That's a total of 450mg of caffeine by 11am. To keep me going I'd add a couple of green tea extracts, each contributing 70mg of caffeine, to bring my daily total to a heart-palpitating 590mg. Then it was time for the gym, where I'd replicate my morning dose of 300mg before a workout. So by 6pm I would've consumed 890mg of caffeine. That's 15 shots of coffee or around eight cans of Red Bull, and that was a normal day. Often there were days when I consumed over 1000mg.

The average person would experience strong side effects from this, but the gradual process of building myself up enabled me to consume a toxic amount without any obvious side effects. In hindsight, it probably contributed to a low level of underlying anxiety. Caffeine is a stimulant that increases adrenaline and activity of the nervous system. Just like any other drug, too heavy a reliance will result in a dependency, as I experienced.

At the time I knew that caffeine had a half-life of around six hours, so I thought that as long as I took it six hours before bed, it would be okay. Unfortunately I was wrong. If you do the maths, after six hours there would still be *half* that amount of caffeine circulating in my body with the potential to disrupt my sleep. At the time I didn't think thist was an issue, because I could just take a bunch of relaxants to try and fast-track the process of falling asleep. Remember, falling asleep at the right time is only half of the battle. Sleep quality will suffer immensely with caffeine still in your system. In other words, your sleep will be worse without you even realising it.

It's worth noting that some people with a particular gene (CYP1A2) can have varied rates of caffeine metabolism. Hence, why some people can consume caffeine later in the day than others and *supposedly* sleep just fine (when tested, subjects consuming caffeine prior to sleep reported to sleep well, yet showed a 20 per cent reduction in deep sleep).

How caffeine works is actually quite interesting. The more time you spend awake, the more your body's internal 'sleep pressure' builds. In a healthy individual this would result in feelings of wakefulness, followed by drowsiness after being awake for many hours. Caffeine simply slides in and blocks the receptor for the chemical signalling sleep pressure, known as adenosine, thus keeping you awake and alert. The longer you are awake, the more adenosine builds. Pumping in more caffeine will only delay the inevitable 'crash' that occurs as the excess adenosine floods the brain. If you habitually experience an afternoon crash that begs for another coffee, consider delaying your first cup until at least 90 minutes after waking. This will give your brain enough time to clear out the adenosine and allow for drowsiness in the evening instead of a crash in the afternoon.

It's not too hard to see how a drug like caffeine could disrupt sleep, not to mention how any other stimulants might act. In all honesty, though, I am still an over-consumer of caffeine. However, I have limited the amount I drink and the timeframe I drink it in. In fact, creating my own pre-workout meant that I have an essentially unlimited supply of caffeine at my fingertips, so either I'll have to enforce some form of restriction … or I'll have a heart attack at 27. I went with the former and at the time of writing I consume no more than 300mg in a day and I do so before midday. This gives me caffeine for my morning work and energy for my training session, and then gives my body enough time to remove the drug so it doesn't affect my sleep.

A rule of thumb I use is to limit caffeine in the 10 hours before bed. When I do this I sleep like a baby doll. I say doll, as they're technically not awake constantly, and I'm fairly certain real babies need to get together and collectively address their horrible sleep quality.

Caffeine isn't the only thing disrupting sleep patterns and negatively impacting sleep quality. A variety of other factors also play a role, such as irregular circadian rhythms, underlying health conditions or drugs and alcohol. Tackling the low hanging fruit first: avoid drugs or alcohol if possible. Contrary to popular belief, alcohol is not the sleep aid it's made out to be. According to Matthew Walker (professor and author of *Why We Sleep*), alcohol is not a sleep aid but more of a sedative. It might fast-track unconsciousness, but it makes our sleep more fragmented and reduces REM sleep, which disrupts memory consolidation.[4] Admittedly, alcohol's disastrous effect on memory should come as no surprise to anyone who has ever woken up after a night out with no idea what happened, how they got home and why they have a tiger in the living room.

My general advice would be to get metabolically healthier. Eat well, lose weight and exercise regularly. That can potentially help to prevent sleep disruptions such as sleep apnea. Unfortunately, due to other factors, some people will still suffer from sleep apnea despite sitting at a healthy body weight. My dad, for example, has suffered from sleep apnea for years, and he is essentially shredded. He has to rely on other methods such as mouth guards, CPAP machines or my mum verbally abusing him the next day for his snores.

Apneas aside, most people would benefit from optimising their circadian rhythm. It's quite hard to summarise in a paragraph, but I'll do my best, drawing from a book I've read on the subject. (The book is called *The Circadian Code*, by Dr Panda. That's a person by the way, not a highly intelligent bear.) The circadian rhythm is your body's internal clock. It triggers cascades of physiological changes and behaviours.[5] It's surprisingly accurate. Have you ever woken up moments before your alarm goes off, wondering what kind of witchcraft caused such an event? Thankfully it's not 1563, and instead of burning you at the stake, we figured out that it's due to a rising protein called PER that increases to promote wakefulness at the time you usually rise for the day.

As accurate as it may be, the body's clock needs some consistency. You can't fly across the country every second day and play 'guess the time' with your body; it would be a futile and expensive activity.

To maintain and optimise a healthy circadian rhythm, you can do a few things daily. First, as soon as you can upon waking, get 20 minutes of light exposure. This will directly signal to your body that it is morning through shutting off melatonin, the primary hormone responsible for sleep. If you live in a place where it's dark until 11am, you can use bright white LEDs if you want to get serious about optimising your circadian rhythm – or you could just move closer to where the sun actually shines.

Just as light acts as a cue in the morning, it also does in the evening. Bright blue lights in the evening will disrupt your schedule. Aim to minimise screens at night to allow the increase in melatonin to shift your body into drowsiness and then sleep.

Once you have an optimal routine for light exposure, you'll then need to eat at regular times. Your body's internal clock will then adjust hunger hormones to that approximate time to accommodate your chosen feeding windows. This is why, if you eat breakfast, you tend to get hungry in the mornings; your body will release the hunger hormone ghrelin at around the same time each day. Conversely, if you want to try fasting, you just need to push your eating window out long enough to convince your body to secrete ghrelin later instead of earlier (this typically takes a couple of weeks, see chapter 17).

Eating too close to bedtime has been seen to disrupt sleep, so I'd recommend having your last meal around three hours before you plan to nod off.

Exercise can be used to promote the health of our sleep-and-waking schedule, as well as a consistent bedtime. Funnily enough, the circadian rhythm relies on rhythms and consistency, so if you can implement a schedule and stick to it, your body will love you for it.

Reducing one of the most important activities in our lives to one chapter doesn't do it justice. But for reductionism's sake I'm going to summarise it as much as I possibly can. If you want to prioritise your sleep: wake up and see sunlight. Exercise. Eat well. Limit the time and amount of caffeine. Avoid drugs and alcohol. Eat at regular intervals. Avoid bright screens at night. Don't eat too close to bedtime. Don't be a witch in 15th-century Scotland.

**DO THIS:** Write down your new evening routine. Eliminate the habits you think might be disrupting your sleep and add in some new ones you'd like to try. Try this routine for a week and take note of your sleep quality and resulting daily mood.

# 13

# The mental hack to effective goal setting

Considering the fact that I made a name for myself as a fitness influencer, it might be hard to picture a chubby young Zac jogging up the street and vomiting in a bush after no more than 200 metres. But to me, the memory is as clear as yesterday's workout.

I was 13, with myriad insecurities about my body image, self-esteem and body fat. The goal of having a six pack was actually out of the question as I believed (like most chubby kids) that it was impossible. However, I did possess a goal to look good in clothes and feel 'skinnier'. So, following my brother's lead, I decided to change my diet and took up running.

On the first day of my newly adopted daily routine, Joel and I left the house and began our 2km run up the street. Despite his words of encouragement, I stopped at letterbox 30, heaved my body over my knees and spewed. It was humiliating. I couldn't believe that was where I was starting from, but at the same time I could believe it because my expectations for myself were pitifully low. But instead of giving up altogether, I shortened the goalposts: from 2km to letterbox 30 (I still remember the house).

Each day from then on I had the goal of getting one house further. Some days I did it and others I fell short. But after a year of doing this I was running 10km daily. I was skinny with ab lines, and I felt like a new person. You would've thought that I'd be happy with how I looked and just continue to maintain my new physique, but the human mind doesn't really work like that. I decided to see what other areas I could improve on. I mean, if I could change my body one way, surely I could change it another?

Then I began my journey with weights. Almost every day for 12 years I have trained with weights. In fact, at the time of writing I have completed at least 3060 workouts in the gym. This was never the goal though. My goal was to improve on my lifts each week, maybe get a bit leaner each month or just a *tiny* bit bigger after a few months. I have exceeded my dream physique by an incredible amount and I can only credit this to the attitude of goal setting.

When most people think of goal setting, it's usually in particular circumstances. One is a new beginning. For example, the beginning of the year, the first day of the month, Monday, a lunar eclipse, or anything else that holds significance. The second condition is a disdain for the current state and a desire for change, which fuels the thought process. Finally, the most important circumstance is a spark in motivation and increase in dopamine that makes you feel excited and pumped about the journey ahead. Nothing feels too difficult when you're setting goals with heightened dopamine; at those times you can't even imagine what laziness feels like.

The problem with dopamine-induced motivation is that it's fleeting. It goes as fast as it comes and does so exceedingly quick when faced with any difficulties or roadblocks. It reminds me of going out on a Saturday night when you and your mate (or a stranger) make grandiose plans for the future, only to wake up the next day with a headache, depleted neurochemicals and absolutely zero intention of implementing what you planned.

Motivation can be a physiological state of heightened neurochemicals in the brain that makes it far easier to commit to doing something for the future. Then your state changes and it becomes far more difficult to continue. So how did I set my goals and complete them? Well, my relationship with goal setting was slightly more complicated. In the aforementioned letterbox example, I started small and just made the effort to show up. If I showed up to my run then I would complete my day's goal.

Over my transition into adulthood, though, I began to fear goal setting. I struggled with anxiety and doubted my own potential. I didn't want to set goals, out of a fear of not being able to achieve anything, so for a while I ignored the activity all together. A few years later, something in my head switched. I think I accidentally proved to myself that I was capable of achievement and the huge world wouldn't swallow me up if I tried. I went back to my early days and refined the process to yield what I use religiously to this day.

My method of goal setting is solely dedicated to achieving consistency. I don't let huge goals demotivate me or throw me off the wagon, and I don't underestimate the small activities. And this is and has been my process to changing my body physically and generating millions of dollars. Sorry, I just had to throw that in there for dramatic effect: it sounded cool.

First I set an unbelievably huge goal. Something terrifying. Then I forget it entirely. It's important to be aware of it, but I can't let it distract me from the small tasks. For example, if my huge goal is to become a multimillionaire and one of the biggest names in Australia, making $100 today and getting shitty engagement on my new post is going to make me feel far worse and further away from my goal. So I acknowledge my huge goal and I forget about it, deliberately suppressing it in the depths of my brain (a place formerly home to my insecurities and fears, alongside memories of leg days previously gone). This allows me to break the goal down into smaller result-based goals that can be achieved over a few months. For example, increase my social following by 10,000 over three months and generate x amount of revenue. I then break this down into smaller actionable goals each week that will generate the numbers, such as posting one YouTube video per week, posting x amount of content on various platforms per week, sending out x emails per week.

Do you think I'm done breaking things down? Not quite. I finally break those weekly items into actionable daily tasks, look at my calendar and literally write them in there. If I have to post a YouTube video each week, I will put in my calendar the time that I'm going to plan it, the time I'm going to film it, when I'm taking my thumbnail photo, when I'm editing it and of course a reminder for when I'll post it. I repeat the process for every actionable item until my weekly calendar is full of small tasks that will eventually lead me to fulfil the larger task.

Once they're completed, the larger tasks will lead to my completing the huge goal, because that's what my plan says.

Sometimes the world isn't so methodical and you'll meet roadblocks and barriers, and that's when you go back to the drawing board and adjust your plan. In my case, maybe I'll realise that instead of posting one video per week I need to post two, or maybe I need to invest more time into a marketing plan. Either way, I trust my plan to push me further and I know that if I do every small daily task, it is leading me in the direction I want to go in. The best part about this is that every small task is *nothing*. I break entire projects down into bite-sized pieces that I can handle even on my worst – interrupted, unmotivated, complicated – days. For example, the idea of writing a book was terrifying and seemed like too big of a project to start and complete. Yet when I set the goal to just write every morning, I knew I would finish my book before the end of the year.

Writing a book is difficult. Writing every morning is easy. Writing every morning *is* writing a book. Therefore writing a book is easy.

My tiny actionable items are in my calendar as non-negotiables. No human can set huge goals and complete them (maybe Goggins but it's debatable whether or not he is even human). But, as I hope I have persuaded you, by sticking to this schedule, I'm confident in my ability to complete intimidatingly large goals because I can break them down into the tiniest of achievable action items.

This changed the way I felt about goal setting and motivation entirely. I stopped looking for motivation to want to run a marathon in a day, and instead incorporated consistent small tasks into my daily routine that would eventually lead me there.

So, to conclude, here's another example. I bought running shoes last week. Yesterday I completed a 3km run. Tomorrow I'll run again, followed by an ice bath. I'll continue this weekly, add some more frequency and distance, then in six months I'll be running 50km. Alright, that's a lie, I actually hate running even more now than I did when I was 13; I almost vomit at the thought of it.

Still, the point remains. Set huge goals. Forget them. Set smaller goals. Break them down into actionable, manageable items. If they're not manageable, your goals haven't been broken down enough. Put those items in your calendar or weekly planner. Don't ignore my last point. Seriously, put those items in your calendar. Then be confident in the fact that you don't need an intoxicated conversation or a dopamine spike to achieve your goals, you just have to do whatever small thing you popped in your calendar that day and let time do its thing.

# 14

# Four mental skills that changed my life

There is a famous study of young children in 1972 known as the Stanford marshmallow experiment. Essentially, the conductor, Walter Mischel, thought it would be a good idea to tempt children with a marshmallow now but promise them a second marshmallow if they waited for 15 minutes before eating it: either an intelligent study on delayed gratification or Mischel just really disliked four-year-olds. Some of the children gave in to the temptation and others sang, stomped their feet and mentally distracted themself from the toughest decision they'd ever made. The immediate results were obvious: some children could practise delayed gratification, undergoing temporary sacrifice in the present for a larger reward in the future.

The reason this study is famous lies in the follow-up. The children who practised delayed gratification for the marshmallows at four years old tended to have better life outcomes years later. If this is true, then the positive takeaway is that delayed gratification is a useful life skill. The not-so-positive takeaway is almost a biological determinism that implies you're either born with delayed gratification abilities or not, as opposed to the idea that it's a mental skill that can be trained, used and crafted in our favour. I prefer the latter interpretation – it's a mental skill that can be trained. Interestingly, the study was replicated with 10 times the sample size many years later and found that only half the predictive capacity of the original study was explained by delayed gratification, and the other half was economic background. Or maybe some kids just don't like marshmallows.

I began my high school years with behaviour closer to those poor suckers who couldn't wait 15 minutes for the second marshmallow. I'd eat whatever I felt like at the time. I'd give in to temptation and frankly, I didn't like waiting. Today, delayed gratification is one of my most powerful internal skills. Something happened to lead me to this position and it took a bunch of croissants for me to realise it.

Recently I was walking through the airport on my way home from a work trip, and I walked past delicious-looking pastries and several lucky people consuming these croissants, Danishes, Nutella cronuts and jelly-filled donuts. I held back drool as I realised that I was actually more 'jelly' than the donuts I coveted. It was 11am and I was still fasting. Something in my mind told me a croissant would be nice, but I continued to order a black coffee and walk to my gate croissant-less.

As I walked I couldn't help but wonder *why* I so easily said no to temptation. Sure, I would've loved to indulge in a temporary hit of dopamine and flavour sensations, but my mind knew automatically that it wouldn't be worth it for me and that giving in to temptation would be going against the grain of who I am. It would be something I don't normally do and as a result would feel strange. Just as strange as if, instead of walking through airport security, I were to look the security person straight in the eyes and start dancing. It would be the ultimate pattern breaker (and I probably would be searched twice and arrested thrice).

I realised that I had actually cemented delayed gratification into a part of who I am. I'm not kidding when I say I thought about this for a week. I had to unpack why it is easier for me to avoid temptation and delay gratification than it is for the next person. I mean, I haven't had a marshmallow in over 10 years, so effectively the universe (Stanford specifically) owes me around 350,000 marshmallows.

I analysed what I believed about delayed gratification and its relationship with pain tolerance, discipline, flexibility and reward systems. Firstly, I believe that all of these are skills that can be improved, practised, learned and developed. Secondly, I believe that these skills operate in their own looped support network, fuelling and strengthening each other to produce a powerful state of mind that lives as a part of who you are. I realise I may be overanalysing the living shit out of an experiment on toddlers, but just bear with me for one moment and let's break it down.

## Delayed gratification

Delayed gratification can be the sole cause of any success story. If you want to lose weight, build a business, adopt new values or gain anything of value, you will have to sacrifice something in the short term to achieve your goal. These sacrifices could be time, money, current desires or the presence of pain. Most people do everything they can to avoid pain, so this is where it becomes challenging.

What I realised about getting into shape is that delayed gratification meant I had to endure some kind of pain in the short term to reap the rewards later. I would probably be hungry, I'd be tired at times and still I'd have to keep moving forward. Thankfully, I changed the relationship I had with pain and welcomed it. I would blast loud music in my room and bash my shins with a metal pole. Okay, maybe not that kind of relationship, but I knew that where there was pain, there was potential for growth. Most importantly, I tied my ability to endure pain into my own core values, alongside an ability to be patient and delay current desires for future rewards.

That's a superpower in and of itself. If you believe you can handle more pain than the next person for a longer time, you'll instil a sense of unbreakable confidence in your own capabilities. I actually use the terms 'pain' and 'resilience' somewhat interchangeably because their relationship is so linked in my mindest.

So if welcoming pain is a skill, how can one improve it?

I'd prefer to lean on the non-masochistic side and take a closer look at the daily activities you plan to do. To me this translates to reps in the gym and the ability to tolerate the pain when it gets hard. This doesn't happen overnight. I've seen countless people start their set and, as soon as a single neuron of pain signals in their brain, they re-rack the weight and look at me as if I'm a psychopath. Compare this to some of the fittest people in the gym, who willingly search for the pain because without it there is no growth. They know that they have to get uncomfortable and endure some level of pain to change their body. But they also know that this pain is temporary and on the other side of it is fulfilment. When you push yourself beyond what you thought you were capable of, you feel good about yourself. It's like an internal hug from a warm, soft cinnamon scroll.

## Resilience

I recently got my dad into doing ice baths every day. The first day he jumped in, his mind told him he couldn't handle it and he was about to die, and he immediately jumped out. The next time he jumped in, I coached him through it and told him he was just feeling uncomfortable sensations, they would be over soon and to just lean into the cold. He lasted over three minutes and came out on a high. He had just demonstrated to himself that he could, and he felt alive and proud. You can't get that level of fulfilment without pushing the boundaries of your mind and breaking through the limiting beliefs you have about your own capabilities.

I treat ice baths and reps in the gym as tools of mental resilience to handle pain. I consider each second I spend willingly enduring pain to be practice of the skill. After a while it becomes who you are and you are confident in your ability to handle more in the future.

Contrast this with the person who constantly avoids pain. When they are suddenly hit with it, like Dad's first time in an ice bath, they genuinely don't believe they can handle it. Without practice, the skill of resilience can never become a part of your identity. Thankfully I found an outlet to train my pain tolerance and begin to associate my willingness to endure pain with growth in resilience. In the end this was cemented into my value system.

## Discipline

The next skill I added to my value system was discipline. Discipline is like the foundation that supports your willingness to stick to your plan and endure pain through time. Someone who's disciplined doesn't think about why they put themself through pain to achieve their goals, they simply take action. Self-discipline is an important part of their identity. Not questioning or doubting your *why* every day is what discipline is.

Sometimes you just have to stick to your plan of action for action's sake. In the beginning, like anything, it won't be easy, but over time you will start to think less and do more. After a few months, weeks or even days of practising self-discipline, you'll start to like how it makes you feel and the whole process becomes ingrained. It's easier for me to stay disciplined with my gym regimen because I've done so for over 13 years. To give up now would be the most absurd break in momentum I could possibly experience. It would be hard for me to unlearn discipline, because I've strengthened those connections in my brain for so long.

So how can you practise discipline? Through consistency of action. Pure consistency and reminding yourself of your ultimate *why* without ever questioning it.

I realise that it's much easier said than done. It's easy to write, read and follow along, but when it comes to actually doing the thing you really don't *want* to do, it begins to get a little bit more complicated. Why? Because, as I allude to elsewhere, humans are driven by individual reward systems and a constant desire to continue what gives us pleasure and to avoid what causes pain.

Imagine for a second that this current reward system is not benefitting us. A hedonistic drive to eat copious amounts of calorie-dense junk food to experience pleasure, or a reliance on dopamine-inducing drugs fall into this traditional reward system, which fails to take into account the pain that results from a lack of fulfilment.

If we can rewire this internal rewards system to experience pleasure from doing the things that bring us closer to our best selves and experience pain from doing the things that move us away from our identity and values, then becoming disciplined, resilient and able to delay gratification becomes far easier.

I used to have this trick when I was training in the gym. During my hardest, most painful reps, I would reflect on an old Arnold Schwarzenegger quote. He said, 'GET TO DI CHAPPAH.' But not that one. The one I'd reflect on is, 'The last three or four reps is what makes the muscle grow. This area of pain divides the champion from someone else who is not a champion. That's what most people lack, having the guts to go on and just say they'll go through the pain no matter what happens.' Funnily enough, Arnie was right in regards to muscle growth and painful reps. Now these are known as 'effective reps' and are closely approximated to the last five reps of a set.

In any case, I'd hold this thought in my mind during difficult sets and the most important thing I'd do is link pleasure to completing the last three or four painful reps, and conversely link a strong internal sense of pain to giving up. So for me, the pain of giving up early was immensely stronger than the pain of doing those three or four measly reps. Similarly, the pain of not getting in the ice bath or cold shower every morning paled in comparison to the pain of shame and cowardice I'd inflict on myself for giving up.

If I complete something difficult or painful, or practise discipline, resilience and patience, then I will absolutely reward myself for it … with a giant Nutella donut. No, seriously, I will reward myself with a small acknowledgment of how good it felt to have accomplished whatever it was I'd accomplished. I'll metaphorically pat myself on the back (my flexibility doesn't allow the physical action) and take a moment to reflect on the win; to realise that I just did something that aligns with my values and that I am capable. It's a small reward but it feels good enough to drive me to want to experience it every single day.

## Flexibility

So once I've cemented discipline, delayed gratification and resilience into who I am through a conscious rewiring of my own rewards systems … I now sound like a complete robot. I assure you, this is not the case, so allow me to introduce my main point of defence and the final skill to master: flexibility. Not in the physical form because, as I said, I still cannot touch the centre of my back. Flexibility to me means rigidity in the end goal but flexibility in the approach.

Flexibility is knowing when to hit the pause button and enjoy the donut. It's taking a rest day when you need it and it's going out for a nice meal without feeling shame and guilt. A lot of people end up crumbling, after appearing driven and strong, due to a lack of flexibility in their life. Because flexibility allows for balance and balance enables the mind and body to work unopposed and sustainably.

The hardest part about practising flexibility is knowing when to use it. I can't tell you when because it's different for each person. Some people do not benefit from a flexible approach when starting their journeys, because their doubts and limiting beliefs will surface, masked as 'balance', and end up derailing their goals. Skipping the gym once turns into a week off. These people might benefit from being quite strict until enough momentum has been built to properly cement the aforementioned values into their belief system. So I can't tell you when to be flexible. If you want to touch your toes now then be my guest, but I *promise you* that that was my last pun about being flexible.

Knowing when to ease off the accelerator can be the hardest part, but if you practise doing so in small increments and notice the benefits it can have on living a balanced lifestyle, you'll know when and how to use it. Like with all these skills, it comes with practice and it comes with time.

Now that we've covered those essential building blocks of mental fitness, we're ready to implement more strategies in getting your body (and your health) to the best possible place. Let's begin.

# Physical Fitness

# 15

# My very own origin story

As you know by now if you've read the book in order, I wasn't always a fit person. I grew up as a chubby kid with a terrible relationship with his body and a complete and systemic loathing for physical fitness. In fact, I was convinced that I was deathly allergic to running and would go into anaphylactic shock at the sound of a beep test.

I'll never forget the mornings of the school cross-country running and swim days. I would be literally crying and begging my parents to let me stay home, to save myself the embarrassment of coming last ... or worse, having to take my shirt off to swim. (All credit to them, they always encouraged me to go and have a crack.) The sheer anxiety of going to a pool party and having to take my shirt off in front of girls my age was petrifying. I wore rash vests at the beach and avoided the mirror, plagued by insecurities. I never dreamed of being fully comfortable in my own skin.

As you might have guessed, I would eventually realise what my body was capable of and, more importantly, learn that taking control of my physical health could exponentially improve my mental health and quality of life. I built the body of my dreams and turned physical health into one of my greatest passions – and one of my biggest contributions to the world. I have personally transformed the bodies of over 10,000 clients in my coaching program, and I have hopefully helped many more through the thousands of hours of free content I've put out online.

Fortunately, like me, you don't have to be superhuman, genetically blessed or exceptionally lucky to undergo such a change. In order to become the best version of yourself, you simply need to dedicate yourself to feeling great, both physically and mentally. Each one will leverage the other and create a self-perpetuating cycle that continues to reinforce your identity and happiness.

Based on the latest available data in Australia,[6] one in four children and adolescents (approximately 1.2 million) are classified as being overweight or obese, as are approximately 12.5 million adults (two in three). Sorry to hit you with such harrowing figures so early, but it's my belief that we should not accept this becoming the norm. We know that living like this reduces not only quality of life but also life expectancy. We should demand more for ourselves and work to create an environment that allows us to thrive.

There is good news, which is that fat is no match for us. It's a weak and fragile adversary that can be decimated. It took me around 13 years to fully master, so please free up your calendar for the next decade or so – I'll give you a moment to do so now. I'm kidding, of course: you, my friend, are lucky, because I'm about to summarise 13 years of experience of managing my physical health in 12 chapters, turning the battle with weight into a few easy and enjoyable steps. Let's explore them.

# 16

# How to stay in great shape for life

I was ahead of my time when I was a teenager, because I realised that I could change who I was by changing the way I identified myself. Growing up never being a sporty kid set my identity to that exactly. I thought of myself as the chubby kid who wouldn't get the girl, have all the friends or love his body. Until one day, I changed my perception. I grabbed my love handles firmly, repeated the affirmation 'I am beautiful' and marched up to the best looking girl in my class. I pointed directly at her and asked her to marry me.

Okay, so I'll admit that affirmations didn't exactly work out for me, but at least I had my grades to bring me comfort. Academics were my thing and the physical side was not. The behaviours I did every day facilitated this identity too: I avoided physical activity, played video games and enjoyed other hobbies, like creative writing and playing guitar.

It was only when I was 15 that I woke up, truly aware of the perception of myself that I had created. I was sick of the limitations I had established and I had a fire of motivation that triggered a deliberate change in my identity. Prepare for the anticlimax: one day I decided that I was the type of person who drinks juice for breakfast.

That's it. Fucking juice. I'd throw an entire fruit salad in the juicer, add some ginger and down my glass of green health.

I chose this as my first change in identity because I didn't have a clue what else might be involved in getting healthy. I just did the two things that made sense to me: drinking juice and going for runs. As you'll remember from chapter 13, before long I went from despising the evolutionary development of running to actually being *a runner*. I didn't know this at the time, as I had about as much self-awareness as the apple I juiced every morning, but what I was practising back then set the tone for what I would use for years to come: the self-sustaining cycle of behaviour and identity. My behaviour every day (running) allowed me to see myself as being that type of person (someone who runs). I didn't make excuses because there was no other option. A runner doesn't *not go* for runs the same way a bird doesn't go around *not being* a bird.

When, at 15, I lived in a village in the snow for a season, I would be up at 6am, putting on my gloves, jacket and beanie, and running kilometres up the mountain in the snow. It sounds brutal, but it was easy for me because I gave myself no alternative. I had chosen to live the path of someone with discipline, and I did what a disciplined person would do. Soon other people would look at me the way I saw myself, further cementing my identity.

This is how you achieve results in the longterm: there isn't a question about whether or not you should do x or y, it's just what you do. There is no other option. I left my home in Melbourne as a chubby kid and came back a few months later 'ripped'.

We can force a change, we can rely on willpower and we can dig deep and work our way through to achieving some astonishing results. But when the once-burning fire of motivation fizzles to a spark and we revert back to old habits, we are in the same position that incited the change. Motivation is temporary and discipline is permanent.

Instead of discipline, let's use the word *identity*, and consider aspects of personality as our foundation. In my experience, this is the key to long-lasting results and permanent change in your character and life.

I'll break it down in to steps. Firstly, you might want to get started when you're in a more positive energy state. It won't be productive to attempt change when you're feeling down, low, depressed or helpless, because you will be unable to even acknowledge the possibility of it working. You know those days where you feel euphoric, highly motivated and like you deserve the most from life? THAT is the state you have to channel before you even entertain making a change.

I used to read motivational self-help books when I was in a low-energy state, and they used to induce anxiety. Once I practised getting into a positive, high-energy state, I also practised entertaining the possibility that I was capable of change.

So how do we get into that state? We know how. Exercise and movement release a ton of endorphins. Ice baths or cold showers release adrenaline and dopamine (remember that big spiel in chapter 5?) Meditation soothes the mind and releases neurochemicals of calm and pleasure. Do this, paired with a healthy habit that brings happiness (I specify 'healthy' because people have strange habits).

You might want to revisit this section when you're feeling 'up and about', capable and excited.

The steps I used to change myself and adopt new habits in line with what I wanted for myself are as follows:

### Step 1. Identify the type of person you want to become

How can you improve on your current state? What *kind* of person would you like to be in the future? How do they look? How do they speak? How do they feel waking up every day? What excites them?

### Step 2. Identify their behaviour and copy them

This is the most satisfying part because it's very simple. Identify what behaviours the person you want to be must do every single day (for the most part) to achieve the results you want to replicate, and copy those immediately. For example, if they are muscular and lean, they must eat healthily and exercise. If they radiate confidence, they must speak to people with confidence.

Start small, with any step that you can manage. It might mean joining a gym and getting personal training to learn the ropes; it might be having a conversation with a stranger. It doesn't matter the level, because that will always get better with practice. The important thing is the practice itself. This is now what you do. You are the *type of person* who does that thing.

You are the type of person who exercises daily. You are the type of person who eats healthily and doesn't eat fast food. You are that *type of person*.

Don't get stuck on this point with the excuse of 'I don't know which behaviours to emulate.' You don't need to know, because what matters is gaining forward momentum. You know the approximate actions you should be doing, and if you have no clue, five minutes of research will provide your answer.

### Step 3. Reaffirm your identity and remove choice

For this to work, like Santa, you must truly believe in it. You become what you repeatedly do, so when you're about to do your daily workout or whatever new behaviour you chose to adopt, reaffirm that this is who you *are*. Tell yourself that there is no other choice. The type of person who goes to the gym doesn't choose what days they're motivated: they stick to their schedule and put one foot in front of the other. You need to remove the choice to make your life easier. Choice is the death of change, and we live in a society with too much choice.

I've noticed that a lot of people relying on willpower create what I call 'micro-choices'. (Yes, I just invented a word. If Shakespeare can invent the word 'swagger' then I can invent the word 'micro-choice'.) These are small decisions that exist to question the overarching choice you made for yourself earlier. For example, if you decided that you wanted to change your health and vowed to stick to your diet, a micro-choice would be staring at donuts in a shop window and asking yourself, 'Should I have one of those?' Each micro-choice forces you to revisit the decision you made for yourself when you were in a higher energy state and forces you to exert willpower to defend your first decision.

Willpower often prevails until it doesn't. When I was at my leanest, the only way I could adhere perfectly to my diet was through the elimination of micro-choices. If I saw someone eating junk food and they asked me if I wanted any, my gut instinct would be a cold and obvious no. I would almost be taken aback that they'd even ask, because I ingrained into my mind never to entertain that possibility. They may as well have asked me, 'Zac do you want to shave your entire head today?' I realised that if I allowed myself to revisit these choices then the cumulative impact on my willpower would eventually wear me down until I gave in.

By replacing the reliance on willpower with a change in identity, you won't want to give in; you just act in accordance with your best self. For most people, this is like going to work. Very few people wake up and decide whether or not they want to go to work that day. They just get up, because that's what they must do. The option to stay in bed simply isn't there. It's how I easily slip into an ice bath every single morning – you can do this too, you'll see.

The most empowering part about identity is our ability to seek consistency in our actions. People want to be seen as loyal, consistent or stable, and want to avoid being seen as hypocritical, inconsistent or unstable – even to themselves. So the more you act in accordance with your identity, the more you automatically reinforce it on a subconscious level.

That's it. It's truly that simple and you don't need any prerequisites or requirements to start. You just need to identify the type of person you want to become and let the behaviours snowball thereafter. I went from a chubby kid who would never take his shirt off in public to a fitness model and bodybuilder in five years. I did this by taking advantage of the fluidity of identity and our ability to mould this to our liking.

I never spoke about motivation, because after being in the gym for 10 years, I wasn't motivated to train every day. I wasn't even disciplined to train every day. I didn't need motivation and it didn't feel like discipline. To me it was easy, it was just *what I do*. I found it easy to stay in great shape because I didn't pose the question to myself, 'Should I make lunch or get KFC today?' Not once did I question my behaviours, because they were so firmly cemented as being part of who I am. Why the hell would I even give myself an option to change them?

Life becomes easier within these parameters of less choice, because when given the choice, we look for the path of least resistance. Without the choice we just *do*.

People close to you can sometimes be threatened by the shift in identity you adopt. People use each other as objects of measurement to compare and contrast. Diverting from the path others are on, or getting ahead, can make them feel like they're falling behind. Some people will be genuinely happy and supportive of you no matter what. Some people, however, don't even realise they're wishing bad on those closest to them. You may have friends who, when you tell them something good has happened in your life, react with a micro expression of bitterness. And hearing of someone's misfortune, in contrast, can make another person feel better about their own life.

This resistance probably won't be direct but instead will most likely present itself through certain kinds of seemingly benign questions that you must take in your stride. If someone asks you facetiously if you're *allowed* to eat that donut, or if you'd like to derail your diet and annihilate a pizza, eliminate the element of choice entirely and end that line of conversation. Don't respond with, 'No, I'm not allowed,' or 'Damn, I can't eat that.' Respond with 'I *don't* eat that.' (The amount of times I've said to people, 'I don't eat that shit' is hilarious, and every time I hear myself say it out loud it just feels true. Try it.) If someone poses the decision to you, don't even entertain it.

If you nail this, then motivation isn't even necessary to stay in shape. You don't need motivation to live in accordance with your identity. A bird doesn't question its ability to fly.

Except for penguins, chickens and emus. They probably identify as flightless, poor idiots. Don't be like them.

**DO THIS:** On one hand, identify what you don't like about your current situation. Fully open up about the things about yourself you think are holding you back. Write a list of the habits you'd like to avoid. On the other hand, imagine the type of person you'd love to become. Write down what they do on a daily basis and write down how they'd feel every day. Write the daily tasks that this person might do and squeeze those into your calendar. Tomorrow, when you start your new activities, remember that you decided to become the best version of yourself. Trust your judgment, remove the element of choice and replace it with action.

# 17

# My own personal recipe for fat loss made easy

My brother turned to me and said, 'Zac I've been reading about this diet. It's called the shrink wrap and after six weeks your skin looks like it's been shrink-wrapped around your abs. It's what the movie stars do to get shredded.'

Sitting next to Joel in a little log cabin in the United States I took my hand out of a packet of chips and enthusiastically said, 'Hell yeah! Let's do it when we get home!'

I was 15 and had always yearned for the fat-burning secret that somehow the world seemed to know. Here it was, and I couldn't believe that we had finally found it. I could relax in peace and finish the family holiday, consuming all of the new North American snacks that Australia didn't have: cheese in a can, White Castle frozen burgers, assorted peanut-butter-anythings and more flavours of Oreos than I'd had individual Oreos.

We landed in Australia and kicked off our new diet the very next day with as much enthusiasm and excitement as we'd ever had towards fitness. Two teenagers with absolutely no idea began a diet consisting of typical 'bro foods', praying to the gods of Hollywood that we'd emerge looking like Hugh Jackman and The Rock combined. Only our bodies didn't change at all, so we moved on to the next thing that sounded promising.

We continued this process for around two years to no avail, and I'm quite certain I tried nearly every 'diet' ever put forward in the fitness space. If *Men's Health* said you should eat chicken wraps to burn fat, I would eat chicken wraps. If *Simply Shredded* said that fitness models ate every two hours, I would prep six meals a day. If *Diet Weekly* said I should go vegan and burn fat … I would pick up the *Men's Health* again.

You get my point: I tried everything, I even combined the diets, but saw few results. My body didn't change and my stomach remained somewhat flabby.

I'm not sure if back then I was limited by the information available at the time or if I just didn't dedicate my time to learning the right principles, but either way it took me 10 years of research and personal trials to develop a fat-burning formula that could work for me – and the everyday person. As enticing and ingeniously marketable as this sounds, it's basically some science-based tools wrapped in common sense. And by the end of this chapter, you'll have this formula too.

I also have the personality type to take things to the nth degree and throw my entire being into the purpose. I once followed an intermittent fasting + ketogenic form of calorie restriction. (This is a horrible approach, please do not try it.) It meant eating nothing at school, then coming home and breaking my fast at 4pm with two chicken breasts, capsicum, a protein shake, some green beans and a large tin of tuna. I probably ate around 1200 calories in one sitting. I quit after two weeks because the combination of the diet and fasting was so intense and difficult. I'll speak to the benefits and drawbacks of these methods in the next chapter.

Do diets even work? Of course they do. If done correctly, they are an organised form of calorie restriction, resulting in an energy deficit and therefore a net loss in weight. It's quite literally physics. To lose weight, all you need to do is burn more calories than you are eating. If someone with a considerable amount of body fat came to me wanting to get lean, I could restrict them to two heads of iceberg lettuce per day (if I had no regard for their health) and guess what would happen? They'd lose weight. So the general advice is to count calories, eat less and move more. Sadly, this advice is about as helpful as an iceberg lettuce.

Humans are not robots. We can't just *decide* that we don't want to be overweight anymore and rely on sheer effort and blind discipline to get us there. Many try to do just that, and even find success in the short term, but it will only go so far; after a while we revert back to the human beings we are. We have biological impulses that determine our thoughts, and, in the end, willpower alone cannot win. We have to work *with* our brains and bodies, not against them.

I have gotten myself absolutely shredded on sheer effort and discipline. I ate tiny amounts of calories, did obscene amounts of cardio and watched myself get the shrink-wrapped look I sought. Only I couldn't maintain it. I always ended up putting weight back on. My blind discipline didn't help my body and it hurt my brain.

Why do so many overweight individuals report that diets do not work for them? Do the laws of physics suddenly not hold when a person has a high body-fat percentage? To answer, we have to define what we mean by 'work'. Most of us (including my younger self) would see a diet as 'working' if it achieved the desired result: fat loss. Others only consider a diet 'working' if they sustain their new body weight for many years to come.

We cannot ignore the fundamental concept of time. If you burn some fat stored in five seconds of activity, is your diet working? Technically, yes, but what if you then eat six donuts and gain fat? If you are able to act *consistently* to achieve your goals *in the long run*, is your diet working? I would say yes.

In short: a diet will only work if it enables you to eat in a way advantageous to fat loss over a long period of time and in a way that's relatively effortless to the individual. This definition can be used as a benchmark to compare any way of eating. There are literally millions of different ways to burn fat and there is no one-size-fits-all diet. There is only what works best for that individual.

I know how annoying that is to read, so I won't hide behind any ambiguity. I'll quickly summarise what I believe to be the best advice for someone trying to burn fat sustainably and effortlessly. This cannot be fully explored in one chapter and would probably make for a fairly boring read (unless you enjoy reading textbooks for fun), but I'll try and explain the most important points fairly succinctly.

I believe there are a few ways that anyone can make fat burning easier:

- Fast
- Eat a majority of unprocessed nutrient-dense foods
- Practise self-control.

Let's explore these ideas.

## Fast

By this, I mean intermittent fasting (eating only within a certain window of time); for example, eating only between 12pm and 8pm. This will do a few things, the main one being a form of calorie restriction. It can be easier to avoid food altogether than to use self-control to eat less. You know the feeling when you eat one chip and then all of a sudden you have a strange craving for the rest of the bag? It would have been better not to have had that one chip.

I have been fasting for years and find it makes life so easy. I'm always just as hungry at 12pm even if I haven't eaten anything as I am if I'd had 600 calories at 7am. The joy is that fasting is mostly a mental game. The body's circadian rhythm is very smart. If we eat regularly at roughly the same time, the body will become aware of what time that is and signal the appropriate hormones to elicit the response. If you eat breakfast every day at 7am, after a while the body will start secreting ghrelin (the hunger hormone) from your stomach to induce feelings of hunger, which causes a cascade of physiological events that result in your apparent *need* to eat at that time of day. But what is really interesting is what happens after two weeks of shocking the system. After two weeks of delaying your eating window (say by pushing back breakfast to 12pm), your body will no longer secrete ghrelin before 7am and will wait until 12pm to start the hormonal cascade.[7]

The physical hunger side of things will subside provided you stick at it long enough; however, it can be difficult to counter a strong mental attachment to food. Some people will push back their eating window and then think of nothing but food until they can eat. Approaching intermittent fasting with this food-centric mindset will likely do more harm than good and can create an unhealthy relationship with food. You will have to judge whether fasting will work for your particular mindset.

If you want to try and you're finding it hard, you can do it in stages. For example, maybe in your first two weeks you will delay it to 8am, and then the next two weeks 9am, and so on.

With fasting, you can also expect to achieve mental clarity, focus and other physiological benefits to the body that come from periods without food. However, in the context of fat loss, we are mainly concerned with the direct, more obvious benefits of calorie restriction. For that reason, I am not particularly concerned with breaking the rules of fasting. Technically, if you consume any calories during a fast, it's no longer a fast. I often will consume around 30 calories during my fast, but it's never in the form of sugars or enough calories to stimulate an appetite response. Caffeine helps with appetite suppression, so I'll often have pre-workout or a black coffee with a low-calorie sweetener.

So tip number one is to fast daily where comfortable. A 16–18 hour fast is ideal in my opinion. It's worth noting the potential positive effects of autophagy that can be gained after approximately 18 hours fasting. Autophagy is a process of 'cellular housekeeping' where damaged and degraded components of the body's cells are removed and new cells are generated. Autophagy can be achieved through any traditional-calorie deficit but is worth noting specifically in discussions of fasting behaviour.

## Eat a majority of unprocessed nutrient-dense foods

This is where I often have a disagreement with people who are part of the cult of calorie counting. It's really fun to eat donuts, ice cream, sugars and junk food and still lose weight (because you've counted the calories), and it's even more fun to tell people that they can do the same. It's a shocking contrary position to the general consensus that we must eat healthily to lose weight.

I had a period when I was hitting my macronutrients, supplementing for my micronutrients and losing weight eating 'a bit of everything'. Only what I didn't realise was that food with a high sugar content made me hungry, a little bit of ice cream wasn't enough for me and counting calories left me uncomfortably food focused every single day. As soon as I removed many highly processed foods, my natural levels of satiety kicked in and my body regulated my appetite appropriately.

The gut or intestinal tract have methods of sensing what nutrients you're consuming, for two main reasons: adequate consumption of protein (from amino acids) and fat (from fatty acids).[8] The appetite is therefore directly linked to this chemical signalling, as well as to your physical feeling of fullness. This is why you can feel quite satisfied after eating a nice fatty steak or salmon fillet. There is another theory that potentially explains the general population's insatiable drive for food, and that is the protein leverage hypothesis.[9] This essentially states that it is mainly the need for protein that sparks hunger, whether we recognise it or not. Therefore, once an individual eats enough protein, they will be far less hungry than if they ate the same calories from carbs or fats. That is, they have to eat more carbs and fat to get the protein they need.

Defenders of flexible dieting and calorie counting will say that they can eat whatever they want and that it works for them. I agree that it can work. However, I don't believe it is the best method for me or for the many people I have coached. I personally believe that most humans don't want to rely on a calculator or software to tell them what they should eat, and that we would be much better off if we could rely on our own internal body signals to regulate our appetite.

Today, we live in what is called an obesogenic niche; a world full of delicious, high-calorie processed foods that cause us to want to eat more and more of them. Our bodies didn't evolve on processed sugars and ridiculously delicious combinations of carbs and fats. Our bodies evolved on animal proteins and fats, and some carbs from plants. The world would be a much better and healthier place if we had no processed junk foods at all. We wouldn't miss the joy of a sugary treat if we'd never experienced it, right?

Clearly this hypothetical scenario isn't possible, so we must deal with the way the world is today. This doesn't mean we have to embrace it. Just because there are millions of tubs of ice cream available doesn't mean I need to eat one every day. This is where common sense must prevail! I eat unprocessed whole foods for the majority of my diet, to regulate my hunger and satisfy my naturally evolved appetite signals, and minimise my intake of junk foods, which stimulate overeating of calories.[10]

On occasion, when I'd like to treat myself, I will have some ice cream. Why? Because I'm relatively fit and healthy, with low body fat due to not eating ice cream every day.

Don't feed your body junk and expect it to produce quality work. Fuel it with high-quality proteins and fats to keep you full and to reduce cravings for other high-calorie foods, and use carbs appropriately as an energy source. An obese person does not need many, if any, carbohydrates in their diet for energy. It's so simple on the surface but complex when we have to account for each individual and their weakness for donuts (let's use donuts as a symbol for all junk food). But it is my belief that once donuts are nearly entirely removed from the diet, so is the craving for them.

## Practise self-control

You can't surrender all willpower. You won't lose weight, even eating healthily, by eating unlimited amounts of 'good food'. That said, it's definitely harder to overeat on unprocessed, nutrient-dense foods than it is with pastries and ice cream!

Better food choices will improve your ability to eat until satiated, but it's also necessary to practise portion control. You know that your body doesn't *need* a huge amount of calories. You cannot eat an unlimited amount of beef ribs just because they're nutrient-dense and unprocessed. You must use self-control and moderation! For me, I could easily eat beef ribs until I'm full and consume 2600 calories in a single meal. But if I portion out 250 grams of steak with salad and some rice, I'll be just as full in only 750 calories. This is where some thought is required: I'm not going to tell you to eat the 'right' foods and then you can unlock the power of gluttony and eat until you burst while still losing weight. No, just like you wouldn't let your dog eat to their heart's content, nor should you let yourself.

You need to track your food and energy intake, to ensure you eat enough and don't overeat. Start with keeping a rough estimate of protein and fat intake, and adjust carbs as you need.

Aside from day-to-day portion control, you will also need self-control when you seek something 'a little cheeky' (dare I say, 'shit'). If you live in our society today and want to socialise, eat delicious 'non diet' foods on occasion and experience the culinary joys of the world, you will need to practise self-control. This doesn't mean you need to drill yourself into the ground and remove a finger if you eat too many squares of chocolate, but there should be an underlying practice of not eating until you burst. Eat until you feel satisfied and are not quite full yet (you'll soon realise that was the perfect amount).

Eating until you are full and eating until you are no longer hungry are different levels of eating. Be mindful when you eat and be aware how you feel towards food. Don't punish yourself and think of certain foods as 'evil' but be objective. If you think, 'I want to eat this donut but that would make me bad because donuts are bad,' you will demonise them. You'll start to see donuts as a guilty pleasure, only to binge on several of them when discipline didn't prevail and then feel ashamed. Instead, when you look at a donut, think, 'I bet that would be tasty. Only it would probably leave me feeling hungry, tired and wanting more. Do I want that? No, I would rather have something else.'

One day, when it is worth the downside, you will make the decision to have the donut. On occasion, this is fine. And most importantly, you won't have six. It sounds pretty basic, but many people are in the habit of demonising foods because they polarise them: 'good' and 'healthy' versus 'bad' and 'unhealthy'. This doesn't mean you should eat donuts (or whatever occasional

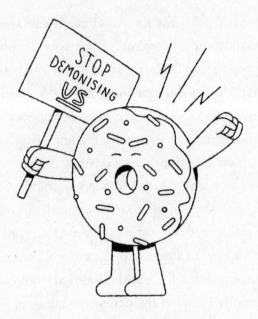

'treat' food) every day, but you can eat them from time to time and not go to hell because your underlying identity is as the person who doesn't (generally) eat donuts.

This section is about eating in a way that's advantageous to fat loss and healthy body weight. Even the most sedentary individuals can benefit from this and lose weight without much physical movement, though daily activity makes it a lot easier.

Piecing all of the nutritional advice together: I will wake up and go without food for a while. When I get hungry I eat high-quality, nutrient-dense, unprocessed foods (to nourish my body and regulate my natural appetite signals). I keep a rough eye on the amount of food I eat to ensure I don't overeat calories for my goal, but don't care too much if I'm out by 5 or even 50 calories.

The result: my abs appear to be shrink-wrapped by my skin and I look exactly like Hugh Jackman and The Rock's hypothetical Wolverine-Stone baby.

**DO THIS:** Delay your first meal as late as you comfortably can. It might just be an hour. Then that hour will turn into another hour, until you can safely 'skip' breakfast time without any negative repercussions or urges to overcompensate. Use caffeine wisely and stay hydrated. Take a mental note of how you feel during the process. If you're food driven and obsessed after two weeks, perhaps fasting is not for you – which is perfectly fine!

# 18

# The truth about diets

Calorie. Deficit. If you strip back all of the bullshit and look at the actual physiological mechanism that underpins every method of dieting, you'd be left with these two words – denoting a negative energy balance achieved through dietary intervention or by increasing energy expended. To burn fat and improve health markers, one needs to consume fewer calories than one is burning. Calorie deficit is at the heart of every fat-burning 'diet', and is also the weapon to destroy every new fad, charlatan, wizard or self-proclaimed expert who preaches their new method of fat loss that 'finally works'. I genuinely believe that if Gandalf was a real, living being he would be doing TED Talks on his revolutionary way to torch belly fat and keep it off, using his new book *You Shall Not NOT Pass a Physical.*

Methods of dieting are a subjective, highly individualised process and people take advantage of personal preference and cognitive biases to sell dieting fantasies. It's like arguing about the optimal morning commute. Person A prefers walking to

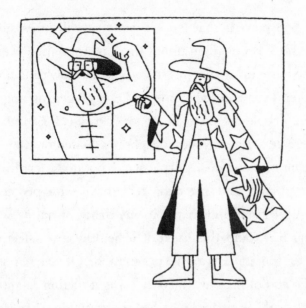

work – they like the exercise. Person B prefers driving, to save time, while Person C fully denounces cars and professes their love for trains due to efficiencies of time, energy and scale. Person D then shits on these peasant modes and takes his private helicopter because he can afford it. There is no 'better way' to diet because each person has their own preferences, imposed restrictions (what type of food and how much is available) and other constraints that they must deal with, such as time, care and money.

When it comes to dieting, it's not all that different. The goal of the diet is to achieve a calorie deficit, just like the goal is to get to work in our example. Many people will find their own particular solutions in achieving that goal; more specifically, in manipulating the restrictions of food choice, time, money and willpower to suit themselves and their situation. And yes, to create a calorie deficit and change the physical state you are in are going to require some form of restriction.

The bad news is that fervent zealotry will often surround each method. People fight about these issues online every day. Allow me to rephrase that just so you can see how ridiculous it is: people literally spend their time and energy getting angry over how other people decide to create an energy-calorie imbalance. I could create a dieting method right now based on the tenets of only eating blessed cows, purple sweet potatoes, fertilised eggs and raw spinach, and sure enough I'd have some people follow the diet, feel great and then join my army of online warriors defending it. Would this make it a healthy and effective diet suitable for the majority of the population? Of course not.

At the end of the day, the only thing a dieting method does is create a calorie deficit, whether the individual realises it or not. Once you understand why and how, you'll be empowered to make your own decision on what you put in your mouth.

## Debunking diets

I'll make this fast and simple. Here we'll look at some of the most popular diets and discuss each one's advantages and disadvantages, and identify which form of restriction underpins it. Most diets are the same. They contain some element of enjoyment to improve adherence to the diet, and a level of restriction to achieve the calorie reduction. If you come across a diet not discussed here, you should be able to use these principles to identify the potential benefits and drawbacks, as well as the restriction method employed.

### Fasting Diets

There are many methods of fasting, such as fasting for a select time each day or fasting for an entire day. Intermittent fasting (IF) allows the individual to consume their calories in a given eating window. For example, someone might have eight hours of the day for eating and 16 hours when they do not eat. This minimises snacking and allows one to feel fuller, having consumed only the same amount of food they would regularly consume in a smaller time frame, thus eating less calories in each 24-hour period and producing a calorie deficit without *feeling* restrictive (for some). Though you'd remember this from chapter 17 because you've been reading these chapters in order, right? And taking notes. And already giving this book a five-star review ... Right?

**Restriction method used:** Time.
**Disadvantages:** Some people become food-focused and hungry when restricting time as a variable. IF also requires two weeks of pushing one's eating window back before the body adapts to the new 'breakfast time'. Some people who skip breakfast overcompensate and overeat for the following meals.

## Ketogenic Diets (Keto)

These diets eliminate an entire macronutrient (carbohydrates) with the goal of improving mood and mental focus, as well as creating a calorie deficit. When you remove an entire macronutrient such as carbohydrates, it becomes quite hard to snack or even eat processed foods, seeing as so many are carbohydrate based. Protein and fats are also very satiating macronutrients and can lead to feelings of fullness and reduced cravings for sweet foods, especially in conjunction with the IF approach when the individual doesn't eat any for a period of time (you'll remember that I found the combination of these methods too difficult, but to each their own).

*Restriction method used:* Food choice.

*Disadvantages:* This can be quite restricting and hard to maintain. I'd be more likely to sell my soul than make a promise that I'll never eat an entire food group for the rest of my life. Sustainability is difficult for some people.

## Calorie Counting (or IIFYM – If It Fits Your Macros)

The idea here is that a person can eat anything at any time of day, provided the macronutrients and calories at the end of the day do not exceed a given number. The exact numbers vary from diet to diet, but the principle is the same. Often this requires the use of food scales and an external tracking app or manual tracking to calculate calories in food and total up your scores.

*Restriction method used:* Food quantity.

*Disadvantages:* This can seem quite robotic and cause a reliance on tracking apps. Without being done in a holistic fashion, people can take a reductionist approach and simply look at food for its energy balance and not its nutrient value, overlooking what specific types of food can do in the long run. For example, a diet high in processed foods and sugars can disrupt appetite signals far more than a diet high in protein and fats. So you can actually be starving yourself of nutrition even though your calorie intake is adequate.

## 5:2 Diet

Fasting-mimicking diets involve eating 'normally' for five days, followed by two days of severely low calories (around 500–600). The mechanism here is that the individual creates a large calorie deficit two days per week, which offsets any additional calories they consume during their five days of eating intuitively. The calorie allowance is weekly instead of daily.

*Restriction method used:* Food quantity and time.
*Disadvantages:* This can promote overeating on the five days 'off' instead of intuitive and balanced appetite regulation. Obsessing over such low-calorie intake on two days can cause unhealthy relationships with food and disordered eating behaviour.

## Paleo Diets

These diets involve eating as our Palaeolithic ancestors may have done. Essentially it eliminates processed food, with the aim of eating in the way that humans evolved to eat. It advocates for an unprocessed, micronutrient-filled diet – not a bad way of going about dieting. By eating 'clean' and removing processed foods, people can experience improved appetite regulation and natural satiety signals.

*Restriction method used:* Food choice.
*Disadvantages:* Unprocessed foods are not magic and this thinking draws on the 'naturalistic fallacy' that all 'natural' foods are in fact 'good' foods. It may be slightly challenging to understand the caloric component of

foods when one believes they can eat as much as they want provided it's unprocessed.

At the end of the day, the most important aspect of any dieting method is adherence. Why an individual adheres to any particular diet is difficult to measure. This is because humans are complex decision makers, filled with bias and unique reasoning. A paleo diet might be delicious and sustainable for one person, yet unenjoyable and unsustainable by the next. When it comes to fat loss, the most important factors are creating a calorie deficit and adhering to that method of doing so. Everything else is just background noise.

I wish I could say which diet is right and which is wrong, but the complexity of individuals makes that statement almost laughable. It doesn't matter what you hear or what worked for the guy next door, what matters is how well *you personally* can adhere to a diet and sustain results in the long run. If living by Zac Perna's praised four tenets gets you results and keeps you happy, then to you I say, 'Welcome and defend our system.'

# 19

# What you eat matters

Before it was normal to open Instagram and see a grown man consuming testicles, the carnivore diet was reserved for a few select individuals and entertaining stories. Or maybe your Instagram isn't populated with ball-eating men yet? Well, give it time.

The carnivore diet has increased in popularity dramatically in the last few years, mainly due to public intrigue and guerrilla marketing efforts. Like anything in the world, attention attracts attention. If you stop in the middle of the street and stare aimlessly at the sky, most people will take no notice and walk right by. However, get a few people staring aimlessly at the sky together and you'll be surprised how many people join in. By the same token, if a muscular man is devouring some nuts (a bull's, not a tree's) most people will watch in disgust. Some will wonder if the man knows something they don't and think that maybe they should partake in the nut buffet. This is what has happened to the carnivore diet, thanks to social media.

In some circles this diet is highly revered, so I decided to try it out for two weeks. The plan was to try the carnivore diet, by the book, and document the results on YouTube. I say by the book quite literally, as I had devoured (not literally) all 500 pages of *The Carnivore Code* prior to planning the video to ensure I was equipped with the diet's 'rules' and any information necessary to support the guidelines. It's pretty simple: eat meat, organs, eggs and other animal products, salt your food, and eat no plants (including spices). That's it.

If you're unfamiliar with the logic of the carnivore diet, the idea is that plants do not want to be eaten and contain defence chemicals to ward off predators (us), making the nutrients we consume less nutritious and potentially even harmful. The logic makes sense, from a vegetable's point of view at least, but I wasn't completely scared off broccoli. In any case, I walked out of the butcher on day one with enough meat, ribs, bones and

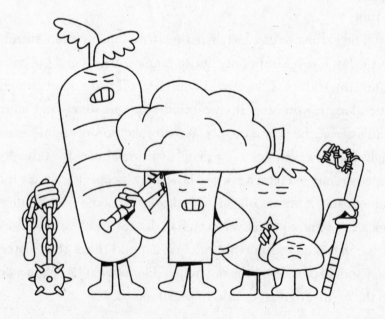

livers to perfectly resemble an actual serial killer. In order to do carnivore adequately, you can't just consume meat on its own. To meet the full vitamin and mineral requirements, you need to be eating organs and bone marrow too.

I love meat, so that wasn't an issue, and bone marrow is a delicacy as far as I'm concerned, but liver was a stretch. Honestly, I think it would be fine if it wasn't punctured with a plethora of holes. Call it trypophobia if you like, but there is something unnerving about slicing into a chunk of meat that looks like it breathes. It wasn't enough to stop me from getting my liver in; I even tried pancreas and kidneys too. I can't say I was a die-hard fan of either, but I could at least swallow them. I did draw the line at testicles … mainly due to fear of asking my butcher if he had any nuts I could swallow. We just weren't quite there in our relationship.

Fast forward a couple of weeks and I was able to relay the results to my channel. In a nutshell (no pun intended), I noticed huge benefits on satiety and appetite, as well as for my skin, energy and focus. Interestingly, the benefits are derived from consuming nutrient-dense and low inflammatory foods. When you eat enough fatty acids, your hormones are optimised and you can think clearly. Protein and fat are both extremely satiating macronutrients. The only drawbacks were extreme dietary restriction, the cost and the fact that my workouts suffered extensively.

The poor workouts were mainly due to empty muscle glycogen. Muscles have a storage capacity for carbohydrates called glycogen, that act to fuel workouts and literally fill the muscle cell. Supposedly, after eating keto/carnivore for a while, your glycogen will regulate itself to a relatively full point. But in my experience, my workouts sucked as my glycogen levels were too low and didn't seem to replenish.

Thankfully, at the time of writing, the carnivore diet has had some upgrades and refurbishments. Fruits are no longer the enemy and some people can even be so adventurous as to include potatoes. My prediction is that the whole movement is undergoing a rebrand from the carnivore diet to either the ancestral diet, the omnivore diet or simply an animal-based diet.

If we all ate like our ancestors, obesity in the first world wouldn't be where it is today. Millions of dollars and lives would be saved. Why might this be the case? Because today we live in what is called an obesogenic niche (see page 123 for more details). Our ancestors didn't have the luxury or burden of being able to quickly grab a packet of chips and discover that they're fishing for more before realising they've finished the entire bag.

We did not evolve to eat processed food. Our bodies evolved to consume food to get enough of the right nutrients to grow and prevent starvation. Humans have been shown to continue feeling hungry until enough protein and fat has been ingested (which supports the success of high-protein diets for controlling hunger and weight loss). Therefore, we weren't ready to consume processed foods thousands of years ago and we aren't physiologically ready for it now.

There has been deliberate investment in food science to make processed food as delicious as possible. Foods are created with the perfect combination of fat, salt, sugar, acid and texture to cause our primitive brain to wish to continue eating them. It's quite ingenious yet scary to think that our definition of hunger has now expanded. Hunger no longer means a physical hunger pang that would be resolved by anything edible, but is a combination of biological, social and psychological drives that make up a feeling of 'hunger'. You don't sit down to watch a movie and feel hungry for some boiled eggs, you want popcorn or Maltesers (or both combined). We get hungry when we're bored, stressed or tempted with delicious foods, due to environmental triggers and social practices.

A huge leap in my own internal regulation of my appetite was understanding when I was truly hungry and when I was just wanting food. I call this the steak test. If ever I was hungry and trying to figure out what exactly I wanted, I would just think, 'Are you hungry for steak?' If not, then I most likely was not actually hungry and instead only desiring food, which is a mental game.

Processed foods aren't made by people, they are made by organisations. Companies with shareholders, earnings reports and financial targets; this is the irrefutable reason why junk food is so addictive. I can't think of a single food found in nature that has the perfect combination of saltiness, savouriness/umami and sweetness, as well as an appetising mouth feel. But I can think of plenty of man-made food that ticks all of the boxes. Humans have shown in clinical studies that they will overconsume in excess of 500 calories when eating processed foods compared to unprocessed foods. This is why it's very difficult to gain fat intuitively eating 'clean' compared to how easily people gain fat intuitively eating processed foods.

The fact that we are surrounded by processed foods means we either avoid them entirely or learn to live with them. I personally tend to do a bit of both, but learning to live with them is probably where the most realistic scenario lies. With that must come food knowledge.

As you would have read in chapter 18, in the context of weight loss or weight maintenance, the physics and end result will be determined by calories in, calories out. If you track what you eat and ensure you're in a calorie deficit (burning more than consuming), you will be on track to losing weight. The next step will be macronutrient and micronutrient tracking, to ensure that you're consuming enough protein (essential amino acids) and fats (essential fatty acids), as well as fibre, vitamins and minerals, to optimise the health of your brain and body.

For most people, this involves quite meticulous tracking. If you want to have some bread or chips, you have to input exactly how much bread or chips you're having and ensure it fits the parameters that you set. Provided this is adhered to, you will lose weight no matter what you eat.

Whether or not this can be adhered to is another story. I'd personally rather eat foods that set my body up for optimal appetite and satiety signalling than those designed to leave me wanting more. It's easier for me to eat a steak with potato and fruit and be done with it, than to eat a burger with a Coke and exactly twelve fries. One meal will keep me satiated and the other will keep me in the mood for eating. However, I'm not a robot or a cave dweller, and will often go out for meals and eat something completely processed. I just have to be switched on and mentally assess when I should stop eating instead of waiting until I lose the *desire* to eat.

The sad reality is that living in today's world you will always need to perform some mental work or restriction when it comes to food. I enjoy a combination of ancestral dieting, calorie counting and intermittent fasting to control what I eat. I fast until around 1pm because I rarely wake up hungry (if I do it's never true hunger and instead just a mental desire to eat). Then I consume 90 per cent of my daily calories from unprocessed or minimally processed foods: animal products, fruit, vegetables and some grains such as rice. Due to the fasting component and food choices, I have already prepared my body not to overeat. It's very difficult to eat thousands of calories of chicken and steak in a small timeframe. If I started my day with a sugary yoghurt and muffin, I'd feel hungrier than if I'd never eaten at all (due to the hunger-inducing effects of high blood glucose with a nutrient poor low-volume meal). For the remaining 10 per cent of my calories I will use some mental restraint and basic maths to decide what kind of processed foods I would like and how much I should consume. For me, this might mean a splash of sauce on a meal or eating a controlled amount of something sweet.

It is my belief that if you push the scale too far in one direction, it will always push back in the other. If you restrict too hard on food choices, you will crave the forbidden foods. If you restrict too much on food quantities, you will feel like you never have enough. So be mindful when setting up your diet to balance every restriction to suit you as best as you can.

As you know, I have personally tried many diets. More importantly, I have devoutly studied these diets. Every dieting method I have tried, I've researched the supposed benefits as well as any potential limitations or false claims.

The keto diet taught me the satiating property of fats and how much I'll crave carbs if I eliminate them. The high-protein diet taught me how satiating protein was: increase your protein intake is often my first point of instruction for new clients wanting to lose weight. Intermittent fasting shone a light on the mental focus that can be gained during a fast and the fact that my body wasn't actually as hungry as I thought it was. Calorie and macronutrient tracking (aka IIFYM) taught me that I could lose weight eating unconventional 'diet' foods, yet it also proved to be mentally taxing for me to track everything daily and chronically restrict food amounts. The carnivore diet taught me the value of eating minimally processed foods for optimal health and appetite regulation. It also taught me that grown men can suck balls online while giving dietary advice, and get paid for it.

**DO THIS:** Practise for the next week consuming a majority of 'ancestral' foods. Ensure at least 90 per cent of your calories are unprocessed whole foods and take notice of how you feel mentally and physically, your appetite, skin health, mood and energy levels.

# 20

# The answer to stubborn fat

When I was younger, I was convinced that I had been born without abs. I remember being 14, grabbing my belly fat and, like any victim in a disappointing shark movie, wondering what might be lurking beneath. Thankfully, it turned out to be a set of abdominal muscles after all. I'd just never seen them before.

My whole life I've had a genetic predisposition to storing fat around my midsection. Most males can attest to this, while females tend to store it around the lower body region. Then you have some guys who never store fat on their stomach and are lean year-round, no matter how many chocolates, cakes or croissants they enjoy. I never wish badly on anyone, but those guys seriously tempt me.

Saltiness aside, the point that I'm trying to make is that everyone has an individual genetic makeup that dictates where their bodies will store fat and how much fat they will store. For me, as I said, it was always around my midsection. My stomach will be the first place I store fat and the last place I'll burn it from. This makes using my stomach as the sole measurement of my body fat percentage quite unreliable, because I'll feel overweight even when I'm not. For example, if I'm 15 per cent body fat (with most of it being stored on my midsection) and my friend Matt is 15 per cent body fat (with his fat dispersed evenly over his whole body), Matt will have abs and I will not. So technically neither one is leaner, only Matt looks leaner.

In any case, this lovely predisposition led me to trying all kinds of weird processes to rid myself of my winter weight. One involved a cream that smelled like fish, which was supposed to assist in burning stubborn fat. I'd apply it liberally to my belly every morning when I was competing in bodybuilding. Who knows if it did anything, but even if it did I wouldn't do that ever again. Imagine rubbing a brown cream onto your stomach so you could smell like fish. Not ideal. It gave my brother an

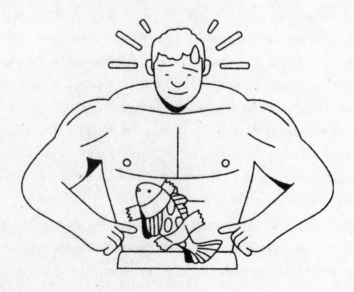

ingenious idea for my new nickname: Fishgoots (fish guts). He'd scream it at me every morning.

Did I finally remove all of my belly fat? I'd say so. But I was consuming less than 1500 calories per day, with hours of cardio, and the rest of my body had zero fat on it. I had feathers in my quads and back yet I could still pinch some belly fat. To get my six-pack-for-summer shredded abs, I needed disgustingly low body fat. I became used to getting myself as emaciated as possible.

The reality is, you can't choose where your body stores fat. As I said, it's a normal genetic predisposition to store fat in a particular location. Some people get a chubby face first, while others get thick legs. You can't really influence this, outside of a few cases that are strictly hormonal or dietary. For example, men with excessively high oestrogen will store fat in their chest area. This can be minimised by chatting to your doctor about correcting the imbalance, as well as natural supplements and dietary habits. (Research suggests that cruciferous vegetables such as broccoli can help, in addition to some supplements. Always do your own research and consult with your doctor before taking anything!) A dietary example would be how middle-aged people in particular tend to store a high proportion of fat around their stomachs, giving them the 'pot-belly' look. This can be due to a diet high in calories causing obesity, insulin resistance or another metabolic dysfunction that leads to fat storage in and around the organs.

Looks aside, visceral (hidden) fat is a silent killer that increases the risk of stroke, heart disease, diabetes and various other life-threatening diseases. The best way to identify if you have visceral fat is to consult a healthcare professional, as people can present symptoms differently.

It's absolutely imperative that you and those closest to you don't develop this kind of fat with age. Standard 'belly fat' just under the skin is much less scary and can be removed by a regular calorie deficit.

You don't need any creams, protocols or wizardry to remove belly fat (or any other subcutaneous fat for that matter), you just need to be eating fewer calories than you're burning. The unfortunate thing about this simple realisation is that there is no secret shortcut: you just have to be consistent and continue burning body fat. The silver lining is essentially the same: there is no secret. Just be consistent and trust the process, and the fat will eventually go. That's it!

Occasionally one might hit a plateau in weight loss and need additional protocols. I'll briefly cover these here for those interested. If you're not interested, and are one of those people who consumes trays of pastries without consequences, then I suggest you skip this section and slam your nuts in a door (if you lack nuts, be creative with any other body part). Jealousy aside, this bit is still worth reading. Good luck with the door though!

So what is a plateau? In the context of weight loss, a plateau occurs when whatever has been yielding results (diet and exercise) is no longer yielding results. The body has amazing adaptive responses, known as metabolic adaptations, that try to return to equilibrium. For example, it's not ideal for you to continue losing body weight because, as far as your body is concerned, at some point you will just die. So specific body mechanisms go into action to prevent this. This might include a reduction in your basal metabolic rate (how many calories you burn at rest) and a reduction in your non-exercise activity thermogenesis (NEAT).

NEAT refers to the calories burned without your conscious awareness. If you fidget, jitter, stand instead of sit, walk instead of stand – these are all examples of NEAT. When you are in a calorie deficit for a while, your body likes to reduce its NEAT to conserve energy. You might not even realise it's happening. Take a look at anyone seriously dieting, and you'll often notice they conserve energy where possible by not fidgeting, jittering, standing etc.

Even though NEAT is primarily unconscious behaviour, you can try to combat this with a focused awareness of your daily activity and using tools like a step tracker. Constantly being aware of how active you are in a day can make a difference in the realm of hundreds of calories.

Another mechanism your body employs to keep you at equilibrium is a psychological drive and desire for food that may interfere with your ability to adhere to your plan.

If your body adapts and you hit a plateau, further reducing calories and increasing energy expenditure is often very successful. However, there are cases where doing so would cause distress and physiological harm, and another approach altogether may be required.

Let's say someone has been dieting for so long that their body has adapted to extremely low-calorie intake. Their NEAT is next to nothing, they're barely consuming enough food to mentally function and they're constantly tired. In that instance, it would be absurd to tell them to eat less or move more. They need to take a break to allow their body to restore its function and reverse their metabolic adaptations. This can be done through a 'diet break', where the individual increases calories to a level of maintenance (the amount needed to maintain body weight) for a period, let's say a few months, before getting back into a deficit once again. Usually the person on a break will eat more food, increase their NEAT and reverse some adaptations. When they get back onto the diet it then yields better results because they have reversed some of the adaptations of dieting that were inhibiting their progress earlier.

The tricky thing with this is maintaining a strict maintenance diet without bingeing and increasing body fat too quickly, leaving the person with more to lose later.

Another method to combat a plateauing is a preventative approach. Let's call it a periodic diet break. It involves a period of dieting (let's say 10 days) followed by a smaller period of eating at maintenance (around two days) – like a 'refeed day', only for more than 24 hours. Two or three days of maintenance calories following up to 14 days in a dieting phase has been shown to reduce the impact of metabolic adaptations and preserve fat free mass (muscle).[11]

This makes sense when you think about it. If you starve yourself for too long, your body will want to conserve energy and try to stop you losing more weight. (It's worth noting that this doesn't defy physics. You can't just be in 'starvation mode' and maintain your weight indefinitely. If you continue to chronically starve, your body won't be able to fight the weight loss and you would eventually die.) If, however, you followed some time dieting with some time *not* dieting (the aforementioned periodic diet break) then your body won't think that you're starving and instead might think that there is in fact food available, so there's no need for it to do anything rash.

You don't need any creams, pills or protocols to target a specific area of body fat, and if anyone tells you that you do, you can find the nearest door and instruct them on next steps. All you need is a calorie deficit and time. There are protocols to assist you along the way but it need not be more complicated than that.

Kind regards, FISHGOOTS.

# 21

# How to gain weight (to stand on someone)

Now, my friends, you've been reading this perplexed. Zac, mate, I don't want to lose weight, I want to put weight *on*. Well do I have you covered, and then some. For the low price of this book I can tell you how to gain weight and also make a little cash.

I've received a lot of strange requests online, like cuckolding a geezer's missus (a story for another time), but nothing compares to being asked to stand on a guy barefoot for 30 minutes. He'd be fully awake and instead of an Ashiatsu massage therapist carefully and gently standing on him, it would just be me, barefoot. For 30 minutes. Oh, and did I mention he was offering $4000? In order to find out the reason behind the man-with-ribs-yet-to-be-broken's desire, I did some searches on fetishes to see if this was a legitimate request.

Let's take a look at some that I found in my extensive research. A crush fetish is when the individual is aroused by watching things get crushed or crushing things oneself. Hmm, probably not. What about a trampling fetish? This is where the person is aroused by being walked or stamped on. Getting warmer here. Maybe if we do some fetish maths and combine the trampling fetish with a foot fetish, divided by the square root of the difference between a climacophile and someone who is totally vanilla, you'll be left with our guy.

Even though I thought that I'd figured our guy out, it didn't make the situation seem all that clearer. And for those still wondering what a climacophile is, it's someone who is sexually aroused by falling down the stairs.

So what did I say to the man in my inbox begging to be squished? I did what I usually do and decided to take the piss for my own amusement. I informed him that I weigh 85kg but can get to 90kg if preferred. He replied, '85kg is fine, 90kg is better though. I have held heavier than that before but that is a bit of struggle, I'm 65kg. So you'll do this for me? And barefoot is okay?'

Now if I wanted to make some serious money I would have to gain 5kg. If I was going to go ahead with this plan, how would I do it? Let's take a look at what is involved when it comes to gaining weight.

Firstly, you need to consume more calories than you're burning in your regular activities, to create an excess of energy (calorie surplus). If you want to build muscle, you need to pair the calorie surplus with regular weight training and ensure you're eating enough protein (around 1g per pound of body weight). If your surplus is too large for your muscle gain, you'll gain too much fat and end up killing the poor guy you're standing on. If your surplus is just right, you'll eat enough calories to support muscle gain but not so many that you increase excess fat storage. This equals a happy man getting stood on.

It's honestly that simple! The complications only arise when someone has been training in the gym for over a year or so. After that, the body adapts to the training stimulus and you have to take a more measured approach. I will quickly go over the considerations that need to be made when it comes to building muscle in the long run, and how to make the most money from standing on people.

You'll need to focus on three things: training, nutrition and recovery. Training will be about ensuring the muscles work their hardest every rep of every set. This means focused attention on contracting the muscle every second to yield the most pain possible using the least amount of weight, to reduce the risk of injury long term. Yes, I said the *least* amount of weight. The second principle is to progressively overload (make the muscles work harder over time by increasing weight, reps or tension).

This might sound contradictory, but I'll use an example to illustrate my point. Let's say you have Person A wanting to get squished to appease his fetish. At first he requires a smaller, 50kg person to get the job done. After a year, he gets used to the weight and the 50kg just isn't doing anything for him anymore, so he graduates to a 55kg person and gets happily crushed for another 12 months, before realising that he now requires a 60kg person, and so on and so forth. Person B, on the other hand, jumps straight to an 80kg person for the first year, because he can handle the weight, and then 90kg in the second year. His ribcage collapses five years later under a 130kg wrestler. Meanwhile, Person A is still living his best life under a 70kg average Joe.

I'm aware that analogies usually frame the example in a more relatable manner, but I couldn't help myself. If you read the perverted example again but replace getting stood on with, say, bench presses, it will make more sense. If Person A can get more out of a lower weight (through mind–muscle connection, intensity, tempo and form), they will yield results without increasing the risk of injury, compared to Person B using everything he's got to lift more weight (triceps, shoulders, joints, tendons and momentum). This idea changed the way I saw training, as it made it sustainable to yield gains in the long run (more on this in chapter 25).

Nutrition is an easier one that I've covered in earlier chapters. Focus on eating nutrient-dense foods that don't cause any inflammation or irritation and create the aforementioned calorie surplus. Some people do have excessively fast metabolisms and I genuinely feel for these so-called 'hard gainers'. Their problems are all too real and yet are met with a complete lack of empathy or understanding as they try to put on weight.

Love ice cream? Try eating five tubs consecutively. The cream will coat your mouth and form a lining so slimy and rich that you'll wonder why anyone thought it was a good idea to extract it from a cow. Maybe you're a fan of chips. Try eating 10 servings of French fries. All you'll taste is the old grease they were cooked in and the salt that goes down saltier than a mouthful of sea water. It's painful to diet and it's equally (and arguably more) painful to stuff your face beyond fullness, even when it's competitive.

It's for this reason that I've made many public videos with tips to gain weight. I call them 'bulking hacks'. Bulking hacks are essentially tricks to consume more calories and have an easier time doing so. If you worry about your 'slow metabolism' and fear that you'll gain weight just reading the following hacks, maybe skip to page 158.

## Energy-dense foods

Forget about nutrition for a second and let's just focus on the energy components. Imagine getting all of your calories from lettuce. If you need 4500 calories to gain weight, you'd have to eat around 60 large heads of lettuce every day. Or you could eat two and a half sticks of butter. This is why energy density is important! It's mainly a factor for carbohydrates and fats, where it's essential to consider the ratio of calories to volume in what you're consuming.

Instead of eating carbohydrates that are relatively low in calories and high in volume (pumpkin, squash, watermelon etc), choose carbohydrates that are dense in calories and low in volume (rice, dates or oats, for example). Higher fat foods tend to help 'hard gainers' get their calories in. Adding things like coconut oil and peanut butter into smoothies can add hundreds of calories without affecting the feeling of fullness. A tablespoon of coconut oil can add 250 calories. That's the same energy as two and a half bananas or 35 cups of raw spinach!

## Cooking methods

Another personal favourite bulking hack of mine (not that I need it) is the method you use to cook your food. Cooking the moisture out of food will inherently reduce the volume and make it easier to eat. Picture boiling a large 500g potato. Once boiled, you have a large 500g potato to eat. Now oven bake the life (and all the water) out of that large 500g potato until it emerges from the oven dramatically in slow motion, like Darth Vader … if he was a potato. Only the Darth Vader potato weighs a measly 180g and is far easier to get down.

Speaking of potatoes, a friend of mine once told me that they had discovered a genius way of cooking potatoes. She said, 'I've just been air frying potatoes for hours! Do you know how many potatoes makes 300g? SO MANY!' It turned out she had been tracking the 300g of potatoes (for the desired macronutrients) in cooked weight: she had cooked over 1kg until they shrivelled through the wizardry of her air fryer. This is the reason why I advise people track food in raw weights only. How you cook food will play a huge role in how easy or difficult it is to consume.

## Variety

There is a reason why competitive eaters can barely resist the urge to regurgitate their 60th hot dog, and it's not only from feeling full. When you eat too much of one food, you experience what's known as palate fatigue, or the cooler sounding term, 'tastebud exhaustion'. The theory is that your brain will associate nausea or an aversion to a food that you've consumed too much consecutively. The result is a difference in your perception of taste. Eating the same thing in large quantities will be extremely difficult. All of a sudden, the slightest hint of flavour will be overwhelmingly sickening.

If your goal is to eat a lot of food at a high frequency, this will be a problem. A simple way to overcome this is to add variety to each meal. Instead of eating 300g of rice, maybe have a combination of sweet potato and rice? Or even a sweet coconut rice with honey on the side of your protein. There are many ways to add variety, so follow your taste preferences.

Now that nutrition is essentially covered, let's look at recovery. Recovery comes in the form of rest between sets during your workouts, and also rest outside of the gym. In the gym you're making micro tears in the muscle. Then, primarily during sleep, your body will attempt to repair these tears by fusing muscle fibres together to create new protein strands called myofibrils. These myofibrils increase in diameter and number to give the effect of larger muscles. In essence: you grow when you're resting, so the more training you do and the harder you work, the more you require rest. Not too complex!

Many people continue to train seven days a week and overestimate their recovery capabilities. The result is that they do not get better, they do not get stronger and they just continue running around like a headless chicken (if it was free to roam in the gym). Everyone has different recovery capabilities. Some people work labour-intensive, physically exhausting jobs and would therefore need more weekly rest days, whereas other people sleep nine hours like a baby and manage to train six days per week just fine.

So whatever happened to the friend in my messages requesting I stand on him? Well, I applied all of the above principles and over three years put on a healthy 5kg to crush my dream of crushing rib cages. However, when I searched Instagram to find him, either he was blocked years ago by me (likely) or he found someone too heavy and is now under 80 tonnes of dirt. Bittersweet ending I suppose.

**DO THIS:** Eat enough protein and calories to ensure steady weight gain. If the weight gain is too rapid, cut back on the calories to find a sweet spot that facilitates good training and slow weight gain. Ensure you're resting and getting enough quality sleep to support strength gains in the gym. If you're not experiencing strength gains, then address training (train harder), nutrition (eat more) or recovery (rest more).

# 22

# Thou shalt not out-traineth a diet lacking valour

There's a challenge undertaken by some YouTubers called the 10,000-calorie challenge, involving the consumption of an ungodly amount of food. There are even 25,000 (and up!) calorie challenges, where the eater consumes around two weeks of an average energy intake in 24 hours. As hard as these may sound, they pale in comparison to the 10,000-calorie eat AND burn challenge. The aim of this is to eat 10,000 calories and then burn 10,000 calories the next day.

Almost everyone who attempts this challenge has failed. One day I went as far as drafting how I'd tackle the day of burning. The morning looked like this:

1 hour on the stair master

2 hour walk

1 hour weights session

My excitement peaked as I strategised. I tallied up the energy this enormous outlay of exercise would amount to and got ... 1300 calories. Just over one-tenth of my monstrous daily goal.

My excitement immediately fizzled. That was an average of just over 300 calories per hour, which meant that I'd need to repeat my circuit for *30 hours straight*. While I may have overestimated my athletic abilities, I was fully aware that I couldn't defy the laws of physics and fit 30 hours into 24 hours. I also would prefer a moment of rest or sleep in there somewhere.

Only when I did the maths did I realise that this challenge is absolutely, well and truly not for me. I figured I'd better just stick with the first part of simply eating 10,000 calories.

You might be familiar with the push-and-pull relationship of eating and burning calories, albeit hopefully on a smaller scale. Many people have experienced what I like to call 'post-prandial guilt' after eating something they probably shouldn't have in an excessive amount. These feelings of guilt usually drive the person to do one of two things: commit to the derailing trainwreck and eat even more or try to 'burn off' the extra calories (and feelings) with some form of exercise. Trust me, I've been there many times. Often I'd do both: I'd ride the train until the very last moment before it crashes and bursts into a fiery caloric explosion, then I'd jump off and begin brisk walking back the way I came, counting my steps as I go.

Let me paint a more vivid picture of a binge episode. Either I'd eat something off my plan or give in to some kind of temptation, causing an all-out fuck it mentality that would drive me to eat every single food I'd ever craved in my entire life. Burgers, raisin toast, a box of cereal, almond croissants, a tub of peanut-butter ice cream and enough chocolate to kill someone. Hours later I'd wake up with a food hangover (with the same regretful feelings analogous to a genuine hangover), look in the mirror and feel like I'd already gained 1kg of fat overnight. So I'd starve myself for the day, add an extra hour of cardio to compensate for the damage and repeat the process the next week.

While this *technically* can work, it is extremely difficult and encourages a horrible relationship with food and exercise, where exercise becomes punishment for straying from your diet. You can start to think of food as calories, and movement as burning calories, and disregard the aim of living a healthy lifestyle. This can lead to disordered eating behaviour.

The issue is that people often don't realise the harm done until it's too late and they have a full-blown eating disorder and clogged arteries.

The extent of one's food intake will determine whether an eat-and-burn strategy is even possible. For example, if you were to eat a packet of chips and a few extra donuts, and down a couple of beers, you could offset the damage done by the addition of some serious exercise. If, on the other hand, you ate 5000 calories over your typical day? Good luck my friend! You'll experience the same dreaded realisation that I did doing the maths for the impossible eat-and-burn challenge video. Hence the old saying, dating as far back as early as the 1500s: 'Thou shalt not out-traineth a diet lacking valour.'

I'm unsure exactly when or who first said, 'You can't

out-train a bad diet.' Nevertheless, the simple truth remains that it is easier to eat calories than it is to burn them.

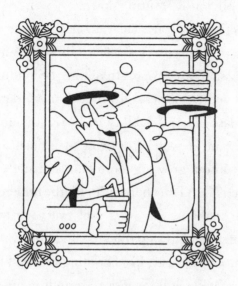

You may have seen scroll-stopping infographics telling you you'd have to run for an hour to burn off a few slices of pizza, or the video telling you you'd need to walk for 45 minutes to burn off a chocolate bar. These often get criticised for only including one of the four methods of the body's ability to burn calories (exercise). In contrast, just by staying alive the average person could burn off that chocolate bar in just a few hours of sitting on their butt.

If exercise is only one component of energy expenditure, what are the other three? Their names are much fancier: basal metabolic rate (BMR), non-exercise activity thermogenesis (NEAT) and the thermic effect of food (TEF).

BMR refers to the energy required to keep your body alive and functioning. Your heart requires calories to beat and your brain even consumes 20 per cent of the average person's daily calories. Interestingly, there are rumours that grandmaster chess players burn upwards of 6000 calories during tournaments while – quite obviously – sitting down.[12]

Your genetics and physical statistics will determine your BMR. If you're a guy over six feet tall with a large amount of muscle mass, firstly: congratulations. Secondly, your body requires much more calories at baseline than a 40 kg woman with low muscle mass. The variability in BMR among populations is quite large and it is very difficult to influence one's BMR significantly without growing more muscle tissue.

We covered NEAT in chapter 20. It's the underdog of calorie burning. The snake in the grass that everyone overlooks and the driving force behind step tracking and fidgeting. It's activity that occurs subconsciously, like choosing to stand instead of sit, pace instead of lying still, or move around on autopilot. These are all tiny contributors to calorie burning, but can add up dramatically over a full day.

TEF refers to the calories burned in the process of digesting food. Funnily enough, you don't actually absorb 100 per cent of the calories in a given meal. Absorbing protein requires 20–30 per cent of the energy you get from eating protein, meaning you only truly gain 70–80 per cent of the calories. For example, if you were to eat 1000 calories of protein (250g of the macronutrient of protein) technically you would only absorb around 750 calories. Hence why high-protein diets are advantageous to weight loss: they increase the 'calories burned' side of the equation. Carbohydrates have a lesser thermic effect, around 5–10 per cent, and fats even less at 0–3 per cent. Most people average all of this out to approximately 10–15 per cent of total calories consumed to get a rough approximate for a daily TEF.

Exercise, then, is technically whatever other activity you do that does not fall into one of the above categories. People often conflate exercise and NEAT because they'll track their steps and then go for an additional walk (rather than the incidental walking you do during the day) to try and increase their step count (typically represented as NEAT). So it's a little confusing at first glance, but there's no real need to get into the paradox of what came first: the NEAT or the egg-cersise.

Now that you understand *how* the body burns calories, you can see how it's possible to influence these components. To go back to our earlier example, it becomes quite difficult to say what I'd *have to do* to burn off the calories in a chocolate bar, considering that the body is constantly burning and absorbing calories in a dynamic process. If I were to eat one chocolate bar containing 250 calories, I'd burn that off through a combination of all of the above.

Okay, but what if we up the stakes to 10,000 calories for a second, to simulate a large calorie intake. There's only so much fidgeting and absorbing and staying alive that can be done to burn those calories. You're still left with thousands of calories, and the only variable left to manipulate is exercise. You'd have to hit it quite hard. Let's say you've done well and now have 8000 calories left to burn in one day. Sprinting for one minute is estimated to burn around 20 calories (1200 calories per hour) so the average person would just have to sprint for 6 hours and 40 minutes to complete the challenge. Compare that with how easy it is to eat 8000 calories. You'd just need to make a single trip to your local cheesecake-selling restaurant and leave with four slices and a single milkshake.

You can go round and round in circles comparing these two forces of calories in and calories out, and I don't think it's a healthy habit to foster. Those who obsess over this equation tend to create a very unhealthy attitude towards food and exercise. With that said, it is essential to know the principle. If you know that eating that big blueberry muffin is equivalent in energy to swimming for an entire hour, you might not gloss over its caloric components when deciding whether to eat it. You'll probably prefer to stick to your meal plan and not tackle any calorie-dense snacks.

It's worth mentioning that all of this is based on approximations. If someone tells you they know exactly how many calories they're burning in a given moment because their watch told them, ask them what the future is like. Because there's no way any current technology is accurate enough to give an exact figure. The only way the dynamic process of daily calorie burning can be measured is through individual trial and error. It's through sticking to a set of physical habits (perceived consistency in NEAT, average step count, consistent meals and exercise) and watching what happens to your body weight. If, on average, your body weight is maintaining over time, then you're likely burning very close to what you're eating. If it's moving in either direction, you can offset the change through manipulating calories in or calories out.

I want to stress again that I don't personally track every calorie burned, because I'd drive myself completely insane in less than the time it takes to burn off 10,000 calories. In my experience, you have to be aware of these components of expenditure, just like you have to be aware of the calorie components in food. You can then use this knowledge as a tool to inform your daily decisions with the aim of achieving a harmonious balancing of the calories in and calories out equation.

# 23
# The truth about balance

'It's all about having balance,' said the large man sitting across from me at the gym table, in between bites of his enormous pepperoni pizza. Like most gyms, this one had a little cafeteria area where people could bring their own meals or buy a pre-made bodybuilding pack that would surely meet the standards of any brand of pet food.

At this time in my life, I was essentially a gym bro. I would bring my pre-workout meal and take my rightful seat at the table with my fellow gym bros. The conversations this table would have witnessed must be in the millions. If the table were conscious, it would be all-knowing and omniscient of everything in the fitness world. It would have heard every conversation between bodybuilders, all the reasoning behind each routine, and every problem one might encounter on the gym floor. The table would be a master of what's known as 'bro science'. In other words, things gym bros say that probably don't have any scientific merit but make sense in their minds.

Some examples of bro science are how protein supposedly develops a layer under the skin, and that's why you must consume a post-workout protein shake immediately after training (not true), or how having more than 200g of protein per day will apparently give you a micro penis (also untrue, I blame my genes). One of the most famous and popular bro science commandments, which brings us back to the aforementioned pizza bro, is one about balance.

You've probably heard some variation on the importance of having balance in your life. As a bro-scientific claim, this actually happens to be true, even if it is often misinterpreted. For the most part, people hide behind 'balance' to disguise their terrible relationship with food and reliance on extremes. Their so-called balance hides their lack of willpower, unfocused discipline and behavioural issues in their fitness journey. In other words, it's much easier to tell yourself 'life is about balance' when you're constantly tipping the scale at either end.

Most people don't achieve true balance. Most people cycle through periods of extreme strictness followed by brief periods of binge eating. Many even achieve their desired physique this way, though few can maintain it. But if they had nailed the balance of fitness, shouldn't they be able to maintain complete equilibrium at their physique goal? Why are they yo-yo dieting, rebounding and ending up right back where they started?

I believe balance is possible, but people underestimate how complex it is to actually achieve balance in health and other aspects of life. I won't pretend to know the answer on achieving balance in all areas of life, because this is something I have never truly grasped. Perhaps because I'm not a monk, because I haven't understood (or even read) the *Tao Te Ching*, or because I'm human like everyone else and aware of my shortfalls. I prioritise work and let my mental health suffer. I prioritise meaningless tasks and say no to simple joys in life that don't seem important but are probably more important than anything else. I have spent years tipping the scale of health at the very extreme ends of disciplined dieting and unhinged bingeing. Thankfully, I have learned from my years of mistakes and many past clients. While I have not begun to grasp the balance of life yet, I am starting to better understand the balance of health. So put down your pizza and bear with me for a moment.

As we know, accumulating fat over time isn't a difficult feat. Just eat slightly more calories than you burn, every day, for a long period. It's analogous to saving money: just put away a few extra dollars at the end of the day or week to see some extra money at the end of the year. The extra money (usually a good thing) here represents the extra fat gain (not so good). And just like you can't

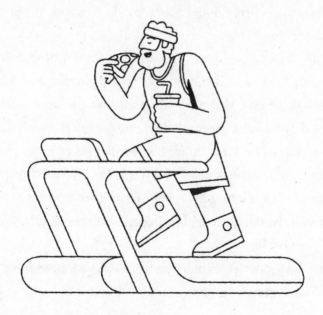

save up for one week and get rich, you can't overeat for one week and look like a house. A large weight gain is the result of eating in that manner for a long time.

Poor eating habits and lack of exercise will tilt the balance in the direction of weight gain. It might feel quite normal to the individual, but it's actually a shift in the wrong direction. Sometimes the shift can be so slight that the individual doesn't even realise until they wake up wondering how on earth they gained 'all of this weight'. To reverse the weight gain and end up at a beautiful, harmonious, balanced point of equilibrium, one has to do the opposite of what brought them to the extreme in the first place. The balance must shift in the opposite direction for a long enough time.

How hard you push the balance is up to you. Some people severely undereat and do enormous amounts of cardio to arrive at an extremely unbalanced scale, resulting in quite rapid fat loss. Others slightly tilt the scale in the direction of fat loss through small, barely noticeable lifestyle changes, producing a result more slowly.

In any case, the important thing to understand has little to do with fat loss and more to do with physics. Say hello to Newton's third law: For every action in nature there is another equal and opposite reaction. When one pushes the scale hard in the direction of fat loss (an aggressive diet and cardio routine), the body will push back just as hard with its own mechanisms in an attempt at regulating the metabolism. If one pushes the scale ever so slightly, the body will push back ever so slightly, which is barely noticeable.

Your body doesn't want to die from starvation, so remember, these adaptations are not a fault of human biology but a deliberate defence mechanism. In a severe calorie deficit, you'll feel hungrier. Food will taste better. You'll feel like moving less. You'll dream about food. It will feel almost as if there is an external force causing these events to halt any further weight loss. The more dramatic your calorie deficit, the more dramatic these pressures may be. Some people can ignore the pressure and push through it using willpower alone (breakups help with this one. It's a common gym saying that the best physiques are built on heartbreak). But before you consider breaking up with your significant other to channel your inner savage, consider the alternative: a slower approach with less internal pushback. The choice is yours.

But what about the long-term repercussions and the path to achieving balance? Let's say you want to lose 20kg. How you tip the scales is up to you, but you achieve your goal and you're 20kg lighter. You now must focus on finding equilibrium at that new body weight.

This process must be slow. The body needs time to adjust to new set points, calm your satiety signals and create a true point of balance in harmony with your body's old defence mechanisms. For the majority of people, this means taking a slower, less intense approach. I've done aggressive diets before and dropped 1kg per week consistently, but I was aware of my body's push back and I had tools at my disposal to deal with it. I knew I was going to be hungry and I expected cravings, and as a result I could tell myself, 'This is normal. This is your body fighting back. Don't give in to the cravings. Stick to the plan. Wait it out.' After a few months of reverse dieting, my metabolism would return to normal levels and I could eat normally at my new set point.

What is reverse dieting you might ask? It's essentially the opposite of dieting. You only consume cheesecakes and milkshakes until you bleed ice cream and sweat chocolate sauce. Okay, maybe not the exact opposite, but reverse dieting begins by increasing calories immediately to a maintenance level (usually a 500-calorie increase from the dieting phase) and then carefully adding calories each week or fortnight in increments less than 100 calories until you're eating enough food. Often bodybuilders will continue reverse dieting to raise their baseline calories so high that their next diet would involve them starting at a higher level of calories. For example, instead of starting their diet at 2000 calories, after a successful reverse diet they may be able to start their diet at 2400 calories and yield great results. Long story short, the goal of a reverse diet is to get out of the calorie deficit as fast as possible and slowly increase calories over time (instead of slowly reducing them as is done during a deficit). This does a great job of signalling to your body that you now have enough food to begin to repair the metabolic adaptations that took place from the diet.

As I've mentioned in previous chapters, there are external influences on your body's set point, such as the food you eat (high protein and low sugar can facilitate healthy appetite signalling) and your daily activity. These need to be taken into account. But the most important thing is to understand the intentional shifts in balance that must occur. This might translate to accepting that a dieting phase is not going to be easy – people often quit because it's harder than expected.

If you've shifted the balance of your health in one direction for 10 years, (towards too much weight) of course it's not going to be easy to do the opposite in just a few short months. If you're happy to lose the weight over 10 years that might make it easier, but who the hell has that kind of patience? I personally would not want to diet for summer, 2034.

So to circle back to the proverb uttered by Pizza Bro earlier, 'It's all about having balance.' The only thing he overlooked – as melted cheese seeped into the crevices of his brain and prevented any higher level thinking – is the prerequisite to have balance and treat yourself in the first place. Get ready to want to throw this book out the nearest window when you find out what it is: the thing required is balance.

Bear with me, as it's taken seven minutes of scratching my head and backspacing repeatedly to give a concise conclusion, but here it is. In order to 'treat yourself' – to go out every now and then, eat some junk food, live a little – you need to balance your mind and achieve more of an equilibrium state beforehand. Otherwise, your attempt at balance through pizza is merely hiding your overpowering desire for food (triggered by the metabolic adaptations of a calorie deficit).

The easiest way to achieve a balanced position is to eat at maintenance calories for a long enough time. The length of time is dependent on the individual, but in my experience, anywhere from four to eight weeks is usually good enough. Once you have eaten at maintenance (imagine the scale at a horizontal even), you will be less affected by the body's internal pushbacks and can act from a balanced position. You can go out and choose to eat whatever meal you want, unaffected by any physical pressures that will make you want to binge or go crazy, and without having to rely on willpower or resort to guilt. Once you're in a balanced position and you've found your new equilibrium, you can easily choose to deviate because you won't be controlled by your cravings.

A lot of people spouting the importance of balance are midway through a calorie deficit and everything in their body is telling them to eat the most calories as fast as possible, and they're searching for an excuse to justify doing so. Balance, to a balanced individual, is not an excuse: it's an educated choice. When I'm dieting and starved, I know I'm not making decisions from a reasonable state, so I'll be a little stricter with myself when I decide to have the odd meal out here and there.

Dieting is a temporary phase to achieve a desired result. No one should be dieting for the rest of their life. The body craves homeostasis and equilibrium. Allow your body to get down to a healthy body weight that you're happy with, and then aim to achieve balance from there.

Achieving balance is not pushing the envelope so hard that you have to reward yourself by deviating from routine and ordering a 45-inch pizza for one. Balance is achieving an equilibrium that is easy to maintain and difficult to disrupt. Do not confuse the two and please do not take advice from the unhinged man eight slices deep into a family-sized pepperoni.

# 24

# How to create the perfect fat loss diet in five minutes

When I was a chubby 14-year-old trying to lose weight, I desperately needed this chapter. When I was a disgruntled teenager trying to get shredded abs, I could've saved myself months of unnecessary work and pain, if I'd only had this chapter to guide my dietary decisions. This chapter is the conversation I have with the mum of three who wants to lose weight but doesn't know where to start. It's the condensed version of what I will tell the middle-aged man to do to lose the gut by himself, without the use of any strict fad diet. This chapter is going to do the majority of the work for you and teach you how to create a diet program that works for your goals.

You just need to work *with* it to ensure success.

## Here is how to build the perfect diet in five minutes

### Choose an eating window

Find a nice, large, preferably north-facing window where you'll be consuming your daily meals … Just kidding, sorry I had to. Your eating window loosely defines when during the day you will be eating. Having some boundaries here makes healthy eating much easier and prevents mindless snacking at all hours of the day (hence why I love the morning fast). Eating late at night and close to bedtime is not ideal for sleep or digestion, so I aim to stop eating two to three hours before sleep. Some days you'll be hungrier than other days, and some days you'll be able to fast for longer. Honing in on your body's natural appetite levels can be hugely beneficial, as opposed to enforced, arbitrary meal times.

### Decide on meal frequency

In layman's terms: how many meals would you like to eat per day? Don't say 10. But when calories are accounted for, meal frequency makes essentially no difference to the amount of fat lost or gained.[13]

Whether you want your calories split into two or six meals, it doesn't matter. It will come down to your daily schedule, your ability to cook and prepare food and your eating behaviour. I personally am fine with two or three larger meals per day, but I know many people who need six smaller meals spaced evenly to adhere to their plan. It's entirely up to you.

I tend to avoid snacking as it's usually an indication that either I'm not eating enough in my main meals or I'm bored. I could become a snacker if I wanted to. I'd just need to practise snacking behaviour for a few weeks, and voila, I'm a serial snacker. I personally find snacking inconvenient and a temptation to eat nutrient-poor foods that are often unsatiating compared to the energy they provide. I cringe when I see people gorge on a 'healthy snack' of apples covered in thick slabs of peanut butter. That's hundreds of calories that could've been avoided if the 'consumer' ate enough good food during their meal. But most people snack for enjoyment rather than due to hunger, so that's also an important thing to note. I allow for one snack per day in the evening due to the universal rule that dessert increases one's happiness. I often have a nightly snack of something sweet and low calorie, such as a bowl of yoghurt, some fruit or protein ice cream.

In my experience, people choose to be snackers. Snacking doesn't choose you. Don't feel like you need your snacks.

## Start with calories

Irrespective of your goal, you have to start with a baseline level of maintenance calories. This is the level of energy intake needed to maintain your body weight as it is. Google 'maintenance calorie calculator' and find one to use as a starting place; it won't be 100 per cent accurate but it's better than guessing. If your goal is to gain muscle (weight), then you want to eat more than your maintenance calories to create a calorie surplus. If your goal is fat loss, you want to eat below your maintenance calories and create a calorie deficit. If you want to do it as accurately as possible, you can eat at your internet-prescribed maintenance calories for one to two weeks, monitor average body weight and use trial and error to find the sweet spot.

For example, if the internet told you your maintenance calories are 2300 per day, then anything less than that should result in weight loss. If it doesn't, then those are not your true maintenance calories and you must use trial and error. To lose weight, you might reduce your calorie intake by 300–500 and make it 1800–2000. For most people, a 500-calorie daily deficit below their prescribed maintenance leveltypically results in around 500g of weight loss per week. Make the call and use trial and error after a couple of weeks to gauge the accuracy and whether you need to reduce the calories or bump them up.

## Plan your macronutrients

**Start with protein.** Now we need to break those calories down into the macronutrients that make up the energy: protein, carbohydrates and fat. Protein and carbohydrates have 4 calories per gram, whereas fat has 9 calories per gram (hence why peanut butter is so calorie dense compared to the same weight in chicken breast). Protein is the most important macronutrient for muscle building, cell repair, muscle preservation and appetite regulation, so we start with that. The average person can consume around 1g of protein per pound of body weight. So a 200-pound (90kg) male can set his protein at 200 grams. This is the upper end of general health recommendations, but I believe it has benefits.

**Move on to fats (fatty acids).** Fat is essential for overall health, hormone production, cardiovascular health, brain health, satiety and more. Whether you prefer a higher fat or higher carb diet is up to you, but as a minimum, fats can be around 25 per cent of total calories and, in my opinion, no less than 40 grams per day. If fats get too low then your health can be severely compromised. If carbs get too low, nothing serious happens. Let's say your fats are now set at 25 per cent of your calories (1900) which is 475 calories. Fat has 9 calories per gram, so you need around 52g of fat. Round it up or down for simplicity as the exact number doesn't really matter.

**Fill the rest with carbohydrates.** If you already have 200g of protein and 50g of fat in your diet, that's yielding 1250 calories. Carbohydrates should come from what is left over (1900 − 1250 = 650 calories). 650 calories divided by the 4 calories per gram of carbohydrates gives you around 160g of carbohydrates. Your macros, therefore, are now 200g protein, 50g fat and 160g carbs. That's your starting point.

Some people love fattier foods more than carbohydrates and so will remove carbs and add fats instead. Others prefer carbs and will reduce fats in favour of more carbs. This is a matter of personal preference and calorie counting.

## Choose your foods

Aim to get 90 per cent of your diet from unprocessed foods such as grass-fed meats, vegetables, fruits etc. These have the most nutrients and will keep you healthier, as well as regulating your appetite. I always opt for grass-fed meats over grain-fed due to the superior omega-3 components found in grass-fed cattle. My favourite proteins to include are red meat, salmon, chicken, eggs and whey. For carbohydrates I go for vegetables, fruit and rice, and my fats tend to come from avocado, fatty meats/fish, olive oil, butter, nuts and seeds.

## Track your food

Spend some time learning how many nutrients and calories are in the food you eat. Calorie-counting apps are great for this.

Here you can construct your own meal plan and play around with the quantities to ensure you get the desired outcome of around 1900 calories, 200g of protein, 50g of fat and 160g of carbohydrates for our male example.

## Monitor yourself and adjust if needed

Your method of monitoring is up to you. I'd recommend weighing yourself daily and taking a weekly average to see the trend. If your body weight is stalling at those calories then ask yourself if you actually consumed only those calories or did you over-eat? If you stuck to the diet and body weight has not changed, then you can either choose to reduce the calories you consume (assuming you want to lose weight) or increase the amount you burn through exercise (cardio and daily activity).

That is why I advocate everyone does some form of exercise. Cardiovascular health and overall health benefits aside, without exercise you can only consume quite small amounts to see significant weight loss. Being active simply makes life easier.

Tracking calories will yield fat loss results for anyone when done correctly, because it is simply physics. It is a tracked and measured approach to creating a calorie deficit – the very same calorie deficit that works for other diets! Where an intermittent fasting, paleo or low-carb approach will place you in a calorie deficit by default (there are exceptions to this), here you can take a less confined and more relaxed approach. (This works great for some people and might suck for others.)

The bottom line is that every diet aims to create a calorie deficit. If there's one thing you remember about diets from this book, let it be this: whatever diet gives you the most adherence and enjoyment will be the most suitable diet for you. I recommend everyone learn the calorie-tracking approach above to ensure they have an educated awareness of what is in food. However, a heavy reliance on calorie tracking can be disastrous, so I recommend you learn as fast as you can so you don't need to continually consult an app or software to try and map out what you eat. Some people can go their entire life tracking meticulously and that's fine. I have also seen many people fall off the wagon, or end up feeling lost without a tracking app (which can in any case be inaccurate).

The underlying theme I keep alluding to here is personal preference. This is why there is very little agreement about the optimal way to diet, because there can never be a uniform personal preference. The key for sustainability is to allow for personal preference but by an informed decision maker. I personally have measured and weighed my food over the years to now hold a firm understanding of its nutritional components. I no longer need to weigh my food, I just look at it. I don't swap out nutrient-dense foods like sweet potato for nutrient poor foods like sugary cereal, because I know the value of the former. I don't need to check how many grams of carbs are in x amount of rice, because I roughly know. I can adhere to my macronutrients (approximately) in my head using estimation and listening to my body to get the job done, and that means I am empowered to change my body composition for the rest of my life.

# 25

# Train for life, build muscle and avoid injuries

If you're in the gym scene, you would've seen or heard of the injuries that come from the lifestyle. For example, during a simple bench press, bodybuilders can rip their pectorals completely off from their attachment point, rendering them immobile and chronically bruised for weeks. After one set of bench presses, these guys look (and probably feel) like they've been stomped on by an elephant or attacked by a shark. A pec tear doesn't need a lot. Just a bit of dehydration, some heavy ass weights and a pinch of bad luck.

I considered myself pretty lucky to have never been injured in the 12 years that I'd been in the gym. I hadn't even had a break longer than one week throughout that entire time! Then I finally did get injured, and realised it was something I actually needed.

Just before the joyous Covid era, I was filming a YouTube video to see how I'd perform on a high-school fitness test. It involved a lot of jumping, running and performing push-ups in 30 minutes of activity. During a set of push-ups, I was approached by an elephant and violently stepped on. The pain was excruciating; I'll never go within 100 metres of a 6-tonne creature ever again. I'm kidding: my injury was a simple pain in my knee from jumping a few times. On the fifth jump, I turned to my brother Joel and said, 'Ahh shit, I think I've cooked my knee from that jump.'

My scan showed severe patella tendinitis, meaning the tendon in my knee was fraying like an old rope. I was so close to blaming that one day of filming, that one jump in particular, and wishing I wasn't so unlucky, until I thought about what I had done in the lead-up to that event. For 12 years I had vigorously trained in the gym almost every day. For many of those years, my leg training involved a heavy weight that was actually too much for my legs. I know this because my legs didn't really grow and I needed fast pace and momentum to complete the reps. So it dawned on me that maybe it wasn't the stupid high-school fitness test that had killed my knee, but instead was years of training negligence.

Tendinopathy requires a very specific and careful form of rehab. You rest. Then you add exercise in very carefully, with slow eccentrics (how you resist momentum when you lower a weight) and light weight. Then you need days of rest. Then you slowly, over time, increase the work. This way, the tendon is given enough stimulus to promote healing properties, but not so much it worsens the injury. So my leg training went from heavy leg press and hack squats with knee sleeves on, to slow body weight lunges at quarter speed. It sounds simple, but I was impatient and pushed the envelope too hard, resulting in having to start from scratch in the recovery stage.

My injury paled in comparison to some of the other possibilities, but it was still a strong enough stimulus to make me reassess what I was doing in the gym every day. I stopped following what everyone else was doing. I stopped lifting the heaviest weight I could at the fastest speed possible, and I gave up wearing every bodybuilding accessory (belts, wraps, sleeves and strap-ons) that I could find. Did I say strap-ons? I meant 'straps'.

This next section might be a little boring if you don't really care about the gym. But for those who *are* interested in training, it could be to your benefit and could potentially prevent you from some injury-induced forced rest.

Before the injury I would use the aforementioned body-building accessories and pick the heaviest weight I could handle for 6–8 fast reps, bouncing out of the bottom and exploding to finish the rep. My form was good. I was going from A to B, taking the rep through its full range and somewhat controlling the weight on the way down. However, my shoulder joints would constantly pull up sore after heavy chest days and my body was always dealing with weakened joints and tendons, requiring an even stricter protocol for wearing straps-ons. I mean, straps.

The accessories made it possible for me to lift heavier weight and the heavier weight made it essential to use accessories. I became used to my body feeling constantly battered and sore following a training session. I stopped shoulder pressing or incline pressing entirely, because my tendons and joints prevented me from lifting any decent weight without agonising pain. So I just skipped the exercise and loaded up on something less painful.

I can see now how this way of training was keeping me injured. The training allowed me to use the heaviest weight possible, which everyone told me was the right thing to do. The principles of progressive overload also stated that I must continue to add more weight or reps (which I would also do). But nowhere in the gospel of progressive overload did it tell me how to reduce the pain in my joints or an overreliance on accessories to complete the session. So I invested my own time and money into learning more about training and started from scratch.

My methodology switched from the heaviest possible weight to using the lightest possible weight for the same effect. For example, if previously I needed 6 reps at 110kg on the bench press to produce a certain level of force by my pecs, I now needed my pecs to produce that same amount of force with 6 reps of 80kg. This meant improving mind–muscle connection, slowing down the eccentric, pausing at the bottom to disrupt momentum, consciously squeezing from my pecs (and not my shoulders or triceps) and keeping the tension on throughout the entire set. In fact, the pain from the 80kg set would last longer and be almost twice as bad as the 110kg set.

After around six months of training like this in every exercise, my shoulder pain dissipated, my joints felt strong and my strap-ons never saw the light of day again. I could also shoulder press and incline press pain free for the first time in years.

I gained muscled from this methodology. But what drives muscle growth? At a macro level, the main driver of muscle growth is the progressive overload of volume. We have to continue to add weight, reps or tension over time to give our muscles a reason to adapt and grow.[14] It's the ancient Greek story about Milo of Croton carrying a newborn calf up a mountain every day until it was a fully grown bull. The calf would increase in body weight steadily over time and Milo's strength would adapt accordingly. Sadly, in reality, a human's strength adaptations can't occur at the same rate of a bull's increasing body weight. If it did, you'd find hundreds of cows at the top of my stairs and I'd be the most jacked cattle herder in Australia.

The principle of adaptation to a constant stress makes sense, however. The body will adapt to a stressor through an increase in muscle to allow the body to overcome the stressor and lift the weight again in the future. This is common sense and was (kind of) understood over 2000 years ago by the ancient Greeks.

At a micro level, the primary driver is mechanical tension. Mechanical tension can be thought of as how hard the muscle is working to resist a force placed upon it, such as the weight used during an exercise. Other proposed drivers of muscle growth are metabolic stress (that 'burn and pump' feeling) causing a build up of lactic acid and muscle damage (indicated by soreness). By adjusting my form to make each individual muscle group work harder during every set and reducing the helping hands of gravity and momentum, I was able to get more bang for my buck on each rep and focus primarily on increasing mechanical tension.

As a result, I'd get more out of less and would ensure that I was actually training hard, without compromising my form or joints in the process. The goal was to slowly increase reps over time with my newfound form, and consistently train close to failure – as in the mechanical failure of being unable to complete one more rep. This is why I tend to train with slight pauses at the top and bottom of the range, in addition to slowly controlling the weight on the eccentric. It eliminates any assistance from gravity or inertia from swinging of the weight or 'bouncing out of the bottom' on every rep.

Focus on the last 5 reps of every set. These are known as effective or stimulating reps, and all match a similar condition: slow contractile speed (imagine the speed of the bar ascending on a bench press) at a point close to failure. To create the most force and tension possible, according to the theory, we need to train under relatively heavy loads or with a fatigued muscle so that the speed of the rep will be slow enough but not deliberately slow.[15] Basically, you should be trying to lift it fast, but due to the sheer effort, it just moves slowly so that a lot of funky muscle-gain sciencey stuff can occur (if you want to read more, search the force–velocity relationship). All of that is what training to failure looks like.

Whether or not you *need* to train to failure is a different story. The closer you get to absolute failure, the harder it is to recover.[16]

If you can't recover then you can't get back in the gym and make progress, and we all know that we need to get stronger over time in some capacity to ensure muscle growth. So there's a fine line between training to absolute failure – beyond reasonable recovery – and just clocking up a few 'effective reps' from each set.

Side note: for those unfamiliar with the methodology of reps in reserve, the strategy is to leave a couple of reps 'in the tank' and not go all-out to failure on every set. While that works for allowing overload and improving recovery capabilities, most people simply don't know where their failure point is and when they think they are leaving three reps in the tank they are actually leaving six. I've always preferred to train very close to failure with perfect form.

In summary: fix your form to make the target muscles work harder and in doing so place less stress on your connective tissue and joints. Train quite close to failure and remember that the last few reps are the ones that are most important. Ensure you have enough food and recovery time to progress over time. Finally, to tick all of the boxes, ensure that you feel some kind of pump and burn in your session.

I believe that changing my training to this new method allowed me to not only train injury-free, but also to target and improve weak points in my physique that I never could have before (back development, calves and hamstrings). Yes, you read that right. My calves actually grew.

I invested literally thousands of dollars in expert coaching to refine my training and fine tune my form to yield this result. I happily give free advice on my social media platforms and offer paid coaching for an in-depth run-down. I think that if this injury happened to me any earlier in my life, I would've blamed the circumstances. I would've blamed that specific thing that did it, such as that one jump. Many others would do the same. The next time you see someone injured from the gym, ask them what happened. I can almost guarantee they will not say, 'Just years of substandard training and movement patterns causing a slow deterioration of my tendons, ligaments and joints and ultimately drastically increasing my risk of injury.' They'll say something like, 'Bro, I rocked up to the gym and just wasn't feeling 100 per cent but I smashed a set of pressing anyway.'

People blame a particular day of bad luck as opposed to accepting the fact that maybe they hadn't been training the right way in the beginning. They attach their egos and their identities to how they perform in the gym and any suggestion to change their form or methodology is a personal attack. Tell a gym bro that his form sucks and he'll look at you like you told him that his mother is a pig. My theory is that plenty of people are injured due to bad luck. We can't deny that. But there is no need to worsen your luck by training in a way that's disadvantageous for the health of your body. If an elephant steps on you one day, that is extremely unlucky. If you get stepped on by an elephant while camping out in the elephant enclosure at the zoo, then you might want to think about how your choices have contributed to your predicament. Or just blame the elephant.

**DO THIS:** The next time you're in the gym, start with a light weight and continuously add weight until you can't get any more reps in the range of around 6–10 reps. Use your mind to make it as difficult as possible on the target muscle. Flex it on the eccentric (negative) and flex it at the bottom, pause for one second, flex hard on the contraction. Keep the tension on the entire time and don't let it come off. Make it hard! Notice the difference in how you feel compared to a regular set.

# 26

# The cardio that everyone should do daily

At some point in the future, when I look back on my life, I know that some of my most treasured memories will be morning walks with my mum. Joel would later join, but for a while between the ages of 19–24 (when Joel was still a full-time carpenter), Mum and I would venture outside for our daily cardio session to start off the morning. Not only was it a form of calorie expenditure, but it solved nearly every problem I had (other than my spaghetti-resembling skinny calves).

Our best ideas always came from a walk. Problems would be solved. The mind was cleared as fast as calories were burned. I never even intended on walking for my mental state; it was just a nice side effect. Now it's common for Joel and I to go for a walk and discuss business ideas, or I'll even take myself out for a solo walk and mull over any disturbances in my mind.

It was during a walk that I devised with Mum the first steps to a business plan for my online fitness coaching brand (after being crippled with anxiety at the thought of it for many months). Joel and I came up with marketing ideas for our business, Slouch Potato, whilst walking down at the beach. You can still scroll back and find the posts on my social media accounts now: Joel floating on a giant inflatable cookie in the middle of the ocean; Joel eating popcorn in the lounge room only to zoom out and discover that the lounge room was actually a constructed set perched on top of a cliff. (Yes, we built the set and yes, Joel always got the worst end of the stick.)

Many other successful people relied on this simple tool for creativity and exploration of the mind. Aristotle, in 320 BCE, would walk and talk as he explored new philosophies, and Seneca would do the same thing in 50 CE as he taught principles of stoicism (you'll remember this philosophy from chapter 4). Then, two millennia later, Steve Jobs and Mark Zuckerberg would have walking meetings.

It's no coincidence that a stroll in the fresh air improves creativity and mood. Science has shown that walking outside increases blood flow to the areas of the brain responsible for learning and memory. Pair that with an increased state of relaxation, forward momentum, unfamiliar nature (nature improves concentration by providing interesting stimuli for the brain without demanding the extra alertness that a walk through the city might involve), and an opportunity for your eyes to focus on faraway distances, and you are on the way to unlocking your ideal state of mind.

It could also be the same mechanism that explains why you come up with your best ideas in the shower. The unconscious thought theory suggests that some tasks are better resolved unconsciously, during down time. Studies have found that analytical tasks requiring strict rules (such as a maths problem) require conscious thought – sitting down at your desk and tackling it head on. More ambiguous and creative problems might be best resolved following a period of downtime, such as walking or a relaxing shower, where the subconscious mind can sift through information and come up with a resolution or idea.

There is a similar method of creativity that I use when I'm having issues solving a problem. First I will write down a lot of the information I have (like a mind map of topics and their underlying issues). I'll do my best to spend 20 minutes internalising the issue at hand and the goal. Then I'll head out for a walk and take my mind entirely off the topic. If I don't come up with an idea during the walk, often as soon as I sit back down and re-enter my previous headspace, I have an improved ability to come up with creative ideas.

We think that our mind is only our conscious awareness, but pay attention to the times when you feel like you spontaneously and effortlessly come up with an idea. Be mindful of the events preceding this, and replicate them. For me, this was a daily walk.

Notice how I haven't spoken here about the physical benefits of walking for health and fat loss. I wanted to emphasise the less obvious benefits first. Aristotle and Seneca also walked their way to 5 per cent body fat and it's no wonder Silicon Valley hosts the annual Most Aesthetic CEO awards, singling out those with feathered quads and shredded serratus due to vigorous walking meetings. Note: these are only personal speculations, but you never know.

Most people complicate cardio, committing to doing something they do not enjoy, and it doesn't last. So even though I personally see the most value in walking (for enjoyment and consistency), it isn't the only form of beneficial movement. You can apply most of the aforementioned benefits to plenty of other activities. Choose a form of activity that involves moving, ideally outside, in an enjoyable way for at least 30 minutes. This could be a walk or run, golf, or public streaking (technically) ... Each to their own. I'm not here to judge.

**DO THIS:** At some stage tomorrow, make time to go outside and walk. Find a new track or revisit an old one, even if it's just for 20 minutes, with a friend or solo. Set a walking goal to achieve each week and take note of how much better you feel after it. Let the positive reinforcement condition your new habit.

# 27

# Small changes
# for HUGE results

So reading what you have so far, you're filled to the brim
with willpower and enthusiasm and ready to implement all of
it! You're ready for me to add even more fuel to the fire of
your burning desire, because that would be the appropriate
thing for the author to do. Unfortunately for you, I am clearly
not appropriate in any capacity so I'm going to give it to you
straight: I'm about to piss on your burning motivational fire.
I'm sorry.

What you're feeling right now is likely only a temporary
motivation, and this attitude can be what causes people to
fail and never truly achieve their potential. Why? Because
willpower, motivation and enthusiasm are based on current
states of the body and mind. You can wake up on Monday and
be so motivated to eat healthily that you stick perfectly to your
diet, run for an hour in the morning and hit the weights in the

afternoon. But after a few Mondays, that fire has fizzled and you're back thinking about the problems you have on your plate other than food. You start to skip the morning runs and only make half of the evening workouts. Then you treat yourself on the weekend. Then, because you stopped exercising, you extend that treat until the next week, until you feel like you have fallen off the wagon and are in the same place as you were before your fitness epiphany.

This is the most common position I see people in. They start off all guns blazing and rely on willpower and motivation to grind through it. Don't get me wrong, many people can achieve outstanding physiques based on willpower and grit alone, but whether they can effortlessly keep it up in the long run is entirely different. In my opinion, it will always be an uphill battle if you rely on grit and willpower alone. Instead, you must employ small lifestyle changes that over time change your identity into the person who *is* fit and healthy year round, not the person who has to grit their teeth and grind for a temporary taste of success.

I'm going to list a few action items I have employed with clients in the past and seen long-term success with. They may seem trivial, but can yield great results and make anyone's weight loss journey much more comfortable. These are your no-brainer bullet points to action immediately. In no particular order, let's begin.

## Switch out your sugar with a low-calorie alternative

It's been estimated that the average American consumes 154 litres of soft drink (soda) per year. That equates to around 60,000 calories per year. If one was to eat at maintenance calories and simply add these drinks on top of it, it would be around 6kg of body fat added. Switching to a low-calorie alternative would save these calories with barely any difference in taste. There is an argument against artificial sweeteners based on studies showing their effect on the gut microbiome in mice. Thankfully for humans, we are not mice, and there currently is no evidence that artificial sweeteners harm the gut microbiome in people. Additionally, there are some highly debated concerns on whether artificial sweeteners are cancerous. You shouldn't consume sweeteners in large amounts, but I believe that it is a better alternative to full sugar. My favourite is stevia.

## Start the day with hydration

I often wake up with a potent feeling of hunger that is actually just thirst. People need to hydrate immediately, first thing in the morning. Failure to do this can lead to a false feeling of being hungry, and also poor health outcomes. After a night's sleep, your body can become dehydrated because you haven't consumed any fluids for several hours. Drinking water in the morning helps rehydrate your body and kick-start your metabolism. Get in the habit of starting the day with a large glass of water (at least 500ml).

## Don't shop when you're hungry

This sounds like the punchline of a joke, but I assure you, this is a serious problem! Research shows that shopping while hungry leads people to spend 60 per cent more than their non-hungry counterparts.

You probably don't need a study to tell you this. How many times have you walked into a grocery store hungry and all of a sudden food never smelled so good? You get a thrill out of buying just one thing, with the promise you'll end up buying highly palatable, calorie-dense, processed food on the promise you'll only eat a little bit, then you'll get home and will be surrounded by temptation. You'll walk past the chocolates every day and have to decide whether or not to eat them. That simple decision, to eat or not to eat, to break your diet or adhere to it, weighs on you. We only have a finite amount of willpower to spend on decision-making, and as the day goes on, decision fatigue can set in. And the more stressed and overwhelmed you feel, the more likely you will be to give in to the wrong decision when you're stressed or overwhelmed.

It's far easier to avoid temptation altogether than resist when it's right in front of you. Shop when you're fed and satisfied, and you'll make the best decisions for your goal lifestyle.

## Eat more protein

Protein itself can be seen as the most satiating macronutrient, as well as containing the highest thermic effect[17] – meaning, it will keep you feeling fuller and you'll burn some calories simply from digesting it. So most people can benefit by increasing the amount of lean protein they eat in meals. The general consensus is around 1g per pound of body weight is best, but thankfully you don't need to get your maths books out: as long as you're roughly close to that range then that's fine.

It's far easier to overeat on carb-heavy meals, containing less protein, and the protein leverage hypothesis suggests that the body will then increase hunger levels to ensure it gets enough protein from other sources. Prioritise protein and watch your body's natural appetite take its course.

## Replace calorie-dense filler foods with high-volume, low-calorie foods

In simple terms, add vegetables to your meals and perhaps swap out some rice for cauliflower rice, or some pasta for zucchini spirals (my Italian heritage would like to slap me for that suggestion). You don't need to entirely swap a food out in its entirety if you don't want to. You just need to ensure you always have high-volume, low-calorie foods to fill up on with each meal. Then you can choose to eat less of the more calorie-dense foods in that meal.

What do I mean by this? Well first let's define high-volume, low-calorie foods as foods that contain a low number of calories per 100g, such as lettuce and assorted fibrous vegetables. Now let's define calorie-dense foods as foods containing more calories per 100g. To illustrate the difference, let's say you have 100g of cooked white rice. In the context of calories, instead of consuming 100g of rice you could eat 1kg of cucumber. I don't know who would actually want to do that, but clearly the cucumber would be more filling. No human being could possibly get fat due to overeating cucumbers, because they'd need to eat around 23kg of cucumber daily.

Your stomach has stretch receptors that directly inform the brain about feelings of fullness, so if you eat until satisfaction from a majority of high-volume, low-calorie foods you are more likely to consume fewer calories than a person eating a giant bowl of pasta. Get creative. Try swapping out a carb source for vegetables, which will give you the health benefits as well as adding variety and balance to your meal. For me, every meal contains a good protein source, a source of vegetables to fill up on, good fats and then carbs where I fit them in.

## Replace desserts with low-calorie options

When I was dieting, I remember creating myriad low-calorie desserts. Low-calorie protein ice cream, low-calorie Biscoff yoghurt, protein pancakes. I would eat my dessert in culinary bliss and occasionally my (non-dieting) brother Joel would taste it to see what all of the fuss was about. He usually hated it because it tasted nothing like the 'real thing'. He compared it to what he was used to eating and his tastebuds rejected it.

For me it was heaven! My palate was accustomed to consuming these foods and not consuming the 'real thing'. I didn't have ice cream often enough to crave it. Instead, I craved my own protein ice cream more than anything (200g frozen berries, one scoop vanilla protein, 50ml almond milk, blend together and consume immediately – thank me later). The less you have certain foods, the less you crave them and the more your taste changes. Experimenting in the kitchen with low-calorie desserts can be a secret dieting weapon that makes you feel like you can have your cake and eat it too.

## Practise removing foods you wish you didn't love

Cravings are largely psychological and differ from culture to culture (for example, the Hadza tribe of hunter–gatherers in Tanzania do not crave pizza or chocolate like residents in Western cultures do). We eat contextually and in accordance with societal norms. To make life easier for yourself, you can reframe what those norms are and reshape the context.

Furthermore, research has found that reducing the frequency of eating craved foods can reduce cravings far more than reducing the amount of the craved food consumed.[18] For example, if you usually eat chocolate on the couch in the evenings, unlearning that conditioned association of couch and chocolate by not eating the chocolate – or replacing it with an alternative – yields better results in combatting cravings compared to simply eating less chocolate each evening. Practise going without fried foods or candy, or anything that you wish you didn't love. Keep a mental track of how much you 'crave' those foods and whether or not the cravings subside.

It's common to allow cheat days on the weekend, when the dieter rewards themselves for the monumental demonstration of effort and willpower in adhering to their diet for six days in a row. However, this means that they are essentially forbidding foods for a few days and then reminding themselves of its deliciousness on the next. The cheat day becomes the norm and the dieting days become the gruelling effort. This makes the 'cheater's' job much harder than the job of the person who enjoys their approved food every day and no longer craves cheat meals. The former is constantly relying on willpower to resist temptation, whereas the latter has no temptation to avoid.

### That said, if you have a cookie, don't eat a dozen

Most people throw the proverbial baby out with the bathwater when it comes to dieting. They adopt a binary approach and think that if they consumed one extra meal or a food that they shouldn't have had, now the diet is over and there's no point in caring today because it's clearly a write-off. You'll remember the fuck it mentality from chapter 22. It's quite similar to the phenomenon of the sunk cost fallacy, whereby a person continues pushing forward because they've already invested heavily in the strategy; similarly, the classic, 'I've already come this far,' and 'The damage is already done' rationales.

When some damage has been done, you still have the choice to do more damage or to cease the damaging activity. Just because you overspent $100 of your planned budget at the casino, that doesn't mean you should sell your house and throw it on red. The dose makes the poison. The next time you fall into this way of thinking, remind yourself that eating one cookie is better than eating two. Eating two is better than eating four, and eating four is better than eating the entire pack. Any time is a good time to stop and get back on track.

### Create a healthy attitude toward your diet

Like most things in life, it's amazing how much of our hunger is in our heads. People who diet and tell themselves they should be feeling weak, lethargic and without energy generally feel that way. Those who tell themselves that they are fuelling their bodies with good food, have boundless energy and feel healthier tend to report feeling that exact way.

Your attitude towards your diet will most often determine the outcome, so you may as well adopt a mindset that will support you. I remember feeling like if I went without food for four hours my body would starve. I could feel my stomach eat itself and turn in knots and I visualised my body wasting away and catabolising muscle. Then I fasted for 72 hours without consuming a single calorie, and by day two I wasn't even hungry. Now whenever I feel hunger pangs, I can tell myself that it's just a gentle reminder from my body to eat. I know it's not starvation because I've gone much longer without food and felt energised and alert.

## Begin with a meal plan

Meal plans often get demonised for their rigidity; however, I've always been an advocate of a meal plan for dietary adherence using a flexible mindset. Personally I am happy eating from a small pool of a few select meals, because if I love a meal, I'm quite happy to eat it often!

Having a base meal plan will assist in the planning and preparation side of things, which is usually the hardest part of a diet in the beginning. Having a flexible mindset means that whether or not you have steak, chicken or fish for dinner doesn't matter, because the meals that you already worked out are similar in calories and protein. An overly strict meal plan can derail one's progress, whereas a flexible approach to a meal plan can make your life easier and remove unnecessary elements of choice.

My biggest issue I found with the IIFYM (If It Fits Your Macros – a definition is given on page 132) method of dieting was I would be thinking about food at all hours of the day, because my meal wasn't decided yet and I could theoretically have whatever I wanted as long as it hit x number of calories and macros. This encouraged my food obsession, and instead of thinking about my work or other things that mattered, my mind would be substituting foods to see how much of each I could eat if I wanted to order takeaway for lunch. Remove unnecessary decision-making as early as you can.

## Identify 'forbidden fruit' behaviour

A fixed mindset of strict rigidity can lead to binge-eating behaviours and an unhealthy relationship with food and exercise. If you demonise a food you are going to turn it into

200

a forbidden fruit. By our nature, things that are not allowed intrigue us and make us yearn for them.

When dieting, if people believe they are *not allowed* foods, they are more likely to binge on them during 'cheat days' and more likely to have cheat days in the first place. Instead, realise that you always have the choice of what to put in your body. Some things are worth it and some things are not. Only you can decide which is which. If your health and weight-loss goals are important, then maybe halting progress and spending your daily allowance of calories on a delicious dessert just isn't worth it.

You can try this the next time you 'slip up' on your diet. Reflect on what you've eaten and understand that you've just set yourself back another day for that meal. Ask yourself, 'Was it worth it?' If it was, then happy days. Who cares if reaching your goal takes you another day? On the other hand, if it wasn't worth it (which honestly it most often isn't), then you've learned something that you use the next time you're tempted. You'll think about the dessert, remember how you felt last time and then choose not to have it; not because you can't, but because it simply isn't worth it for you.

This is why the analogy of money works so well for people when conceptualising calories. You could spend your week's wage on something printed in Gucci, or you could choose not to shop and accumulate savings. The choice is yours. Most people choose wisely; plenty of people could buy designer items but choose not to because they'd have zero savings afterwards. The same goes for your choice in food. You can absolutely spend over your daily calorie allowance on 'junk food', but you'll have to deal with the consequences of weight gain. By contrast, you can choose to spend your daily calorie allowance on nutritious foods and be in a calorie deficit. You always have a choice and it's about choosing what's best for you and your goals.

## Practise self-control and reward good decision-making when eating out

I wanted to include this here because many people are perfectly fine dieting when in the comfort of their own kitchen, but as soon as they leave the house and go into a restaurant all hell breaks loose. They adopt the fuck it mentality. Some people avoid this by refusing to go out and constantly deny social engagements; knowing they can't trust themselves to make good decisions. But there is nothing honourable about refusing to attend events or bringing your own chicken and rice in a Tupperware container to dinner.

It's empowering to know you can make good decisions when socially interacting with friends and family. The reality is, you can always choose something from the menu that is in line with your goals. I personally love the challenge of going out for dinner and deliberately choosing my meal. Just because they have pizza on the menu doesn't mean I need to order it. I will choose the healthiest option I can. If it's a little short on protein, the world will still be okay in the morning and I'm sure I won't starve. Sometimes I'll decide that a particular meal *is* worth setting aside my goals, and I will choose and enjoy that.

The same goes for alcohol. Consuming excess amounts can adversely harm your liver and hormones, making it even harder to stay lean and healthy. However, consuming alcohol in small amounts and being aware of the calories in each drink can coexist with a healthy lifestyle. Alcohol has 7 calories per gram so even with low carb drinks, you still need to be mindful of the calories consumed.

Practising these decisions and rewarding yourself for doing so (with a pat on the back, not a tub of ice cream) does wonders for your relationship with food and your social circle.

### Reward yourself with something other than food

Everyone is different! Some people cannot eat when under stress and others resort to food when stressed. Comfort eating might provide some temporary relief, but it often becomes a crutch and a tough habit to break, and can sabotage one's health goals.

If you tend to seek food during stressful times, aim to identify the behaviour and the food choice, then detach and ask yourself whether you really want that particular food or just the desired comfort. If you can, try to replace the behaviour with something else. Productivity often helps here. If you can, take your mind off the stress by doing something that benefits your life, such as cleaning, exercising, meditating or even doing your tax – it's a win-win. Your habits become what you do and it is entirely within your control to switch out habits that are not benefiting your life with ones that will.

### Go for a short walk every day and keep an eye on your steps

You would have seen the full chapter dedicated to this (page 188). So go on, do it.

I believe everyone has the capacity to make any small change I've covered in this section to live a healthier and happier life. And despite what the cheesecake and chocolate want you to think, there is freedom in creating reward systems outside of food. A huge one for me has been creating and fostering a passion for helping others through social media and ultimately my business. I have managed to turn the simple act of posting a few photos of myself in the gym on Instagram into several brands and millions of dollars. And because you're reading this (that means we're friends now by the way – best friends, even) I'm about to share exactly how I did it and extract some of the pivotal lessons I learned along the way.

# Social
# Media

# 28

# The secrets to social media growth

I never thought that I'd be considered an authority on social media. I feel like I'm always looking for more ways to work with the system, strategise and be ahead of the curve. Yet in 2023 alone I've been called an OG of the fitness industry enough times to make me feel like an Old Grandpa.

So yes, admittedly I've found some longevity in an industry that can be quite unforgiving. It turns out that very few people hang around for multiple years (for reasons that we will get into later). Many are so captivated by the fame of it all that they overlook the enormous upside potential and money on the table if you play your cards right and build a strong career. So how did I do it? How did I gain over a million followers, make a career out of my passion and learn vital entrepreneurial skills?

It's a secret and I will take it to my grave. The end.

...

Imagine if I left a cliffhanger like that with absolutely no answers. Hilarious joke, but I can already see the reviews. 'Great questions, zero answers. This guy is truly an idiot.' So instead I'm going to give you an unfiltered and honest insight into everything I can tell you about my experience on social media. In exchange, I expect a pretty cool review ☺.

I've wanted to pursue social media via fitness ever since I saw that it could be done. If I'm being honest with myself, it probably was born from a superficial desire for validation and to mask insecurities, but it also carried a deeper goal. I truly love sharing my message and helping others.

I believe that to be successful in social media you *have* to love it. Just like anything else, you cannot do it for long if you don't. I spent a lot of time analysing what other people were doing, what I was doing, what worked for other people and what worked for me. I was constantly assessing the landscape. As a result I had a fairly clear game plan even as early as five years ago, before it was even my job. You could say that making a living out of social media was part of a well thought-out, ingenious plan, yet it felt far more like a sequence of random events all pointing to the one end goal: to influence a community of people in a way that makes their lives better.

That has always been my end goal. I want to add value to and potentially change people's lives through improving their physical and mental health.

One motivation for someone's social media growth might be, 'I want to buy things and use internet money to flex on people who doubted me.' Perhaps that reason is just as strong as mine; who am I to say? It may even be stronger. But whatever the motivation, it has to be strong enough to keep you going. In my opinion, giving back to others is the strongest reason there is.

In the language of marketing, if you are growing your own personal social media then you are the brand. Brands are also personalising themselves more and more today – using people to create content in line with their brand identity. So when I talk about growing social media for a person, this can also be applied to companies.

I have quite an overthinking, analytical brain. I'll create random experiments in my head to test the efficiency of anything and everything that I do. This usually ends up with me wondering if the universe contains the real secret to the most enjoyable way to cut and eat a mango without any mess. Every so often I'll stumble upon something that is actually useful, and in this case it was three actionable steps that anyone can use to create success on a social media platform.

For the sake of my ego, let's give these a nice catchy name: how about the Three Truths of Life? Nope, sounds like I'm a cult leader. What about the Three Steps to Successful Socials, or the 3 S's for short? Done. A catchy name isn't important when the actual content is.

In my opinion, these steps have the power to lead almost any individual (or company) to social media success. I can't promise that it will work for everyone, because we don't live an infinite number of years, and probability states that some people sooner or later will be the unlucky ones. That's not meant to be disheartening, it's just the truth. My steps won't work for everyone, but they might work for you and that's all the encouragement you should need.

The three steps can be summarised briefly as creating a niche, adding value and becoming a robot.

## Step 1. Creating a niche

The first step is creating a niche and identifying your competitive advantage. This step is now more important than ever, considering, as of October 2022, the world had 4.7 billion social media users, contributing to an approximately 12.5 trillion hours online. It's a hyper competitive industry with more and more users joining and posting every day. Just as in any other industry, the more players there are, the more need there is to differentiate.

Let's look at the fitness industry. Gone are the days when fitness influencers could become successful with fitness advice alone. Back in 2014, the guys and girls at the top of the social media game just had to have an awe-inspiring physique. Then users realised there were millions of impressive physiques and the standard shifted upward. Now a social media personality needs to create a niche where they can stand out from the overall crowd. This is a good thing, in my opinion, as it allows for expression of individuality and discourages 'personality' based on something purely superficial.

The downside is that you have to get creative, and this can lead to extremes. The rising social media superstars of the last couple of years have proven this. The popular ones are the ones that attract attention, and being extremely different begets attention.

So does that mean you *need* to be extreme? In my opinion, you don't need to film yourself eating testicles or hold a belief so strong that it offends half of the planet to create your niche. But you do have to be different. Think of it from a marketing perspective. You are the product and you need to identify your unique selling points (USPs) that make you stand out from the crowd and give you a competitive advantage. Dig deep: there will be many things that make you different.

The combination of all of your idiosyncrasies creates something that doesn't exist in any other person (unless we live in a multiverse). It might be the fact that you love fitness, have a dry sense of humour and possess a passion for Pokémon. You might then use your USPs to create informative short-form content about fitness with funny Pokémon references, demonstrating correct form in the gym. For example, you might Pika-choose a weight that you can comfortably hit Mewtwo sets of 10 with, and create (hopefully better) in-jokes with your followers. I'm just spit balling here, but you get the gist.

Once you can analyse yourself as a product and identify the things that make you different, you can take a step back and see how they could work together to create content, and form an online personality. Think about it this way: if you were to be successful, how would people describe you to their friends? Going back to the earlier example, one might say, 'Have you seen Pokébro? He's like a gym bro but he's also a genuine Pokémon fan and his content always has some kind of funny reference. It's actually great,' as opposed to '@Gymbro_1457 is just like every other wannabe gym guy.'

There has to be a point of difference and you have to derive it from your unique thoughts, interests and desires. This doesn't have to be extreme or silly either. Some of my unique selling points lie in the intersection of fitness and humour. A lot of my content is educational and entertaining, and sometimes I double down on sketches and funny impersonations because not many people could also do that and stand out. I had to embrace my weirdness instead of copying others and looking to be like everyone else. In fact, I distinctly remember being at a fitness expo in Perth back in 2016 (before I had cemented my brand personality online) and wondering how the hell I was going to be successful if I was the skinniest and fattest person standing at the booth. I was so focused on my physique I didn't even realise that my physique wasn't going to give me success on social media: it was the combination of everything else that I could use.

The bestselling author and social media phenomenon James Smith gives fitness advice in a 'no bullshit' approach. Andrew Huberman educates millions on the topics of the brain and body in ways that no one else has been able to do yet, by making science accessible to everyday people. Brian Johnson constructed his online personality as The Liver King with the goal of reaching a million followers – a goal he attained quite quickly (prior to the controversy surrounding him). He knew he would get there by his unique approach online: as a jacked and shredded bearded man biting into raw animal organs, yelling about the benefits of doing so. Love him or hate him, you have to admit it's actually quite smart.

### Step 2. Adding value

Once you've established what your niche is going to be and how you are going to be perceived as different, the next step is to create quality content. More people are pumping out more content than ever and the standard for content is rising. Current social media apps may have single-handedly shifted attention spans to only tolerate shorter videos. Trends constantly shift the standard of content and as a result we adapt in terms of what content we enjoy and what content we should produce.

Despite this, I firmly believe that content should be high quality that adds value. It's quite simple. People want to be entertained, educated, validated or motivated, and you can tailor your content to these needs. I also believe a lot of people want to be frustrated or angry, which is why content that is 'triggering' also performs well and sparks comments that further ignite growth. Perhaps this is due to anger being tethered to the dopamine system, encouraging people to almost be drawn towards challenges or frustration. I wouldn't recommend pursuing the latter route, as I just don't think it's making the world a better place, but I acknowledge that many successful people online produce negative content and this may be why.

In my opinion, your goal should be to enrich the lives of others. Add value in ways that only you can, in the form of educating people, empowering them, motivating them, or entertaining them or anything else. Then experiment with different mediums: photos, videos, short-form videos, long-form videos, different editing styles – everything.

If your goal is content creation, you need to educate yourself on the best way to create. I developed a hobby for photography and filmmaking, and now I edit nearly all of my content simply because I enjoy it. I recommend outsourcing when the time is right, but in the beginning you might not have the budget for that and will need to learn the ropes yourself. Learn how to use a camera and learn how to edit, and take it from there.

If your message is great but your delivery is horrible, sadly most people will scroll past you. You have to deliver your message in a way that resonates with your community. Furthermore, adding value to people over time begins to create a community of like-minded people who all enjoy your content and message. You can then take advantage of this and bring the community even closer together. Encourage comments and discussions, mention your followers in your content and show them how appreciative you are to have people who support you.

The most successful creators or influencers have communities that can have discussions in the comments with no intervention. Look at any Joe Rogan podcast clip on YouTube and you'll find thousands of comments, with viewers sharing their opinions, joys or frustrations. This comment section feels like a bunch of mutual friends, as they all feel like they know Joe.

## Step 3. Becoming a robot

Finally, you have to become a content robot. You have to persevere, consistently produce and pump out material, and evaluate as you go. It's a rinse-and-repeat sequence of idea generation and execution. Brainstorm, plan, film, edit, post, gather data and repeat.

A lot of people will give advice about social media that boils down to mere consistency, but if you're consistently putting out shitty content with no self-awareness, you're consistently going to be performing horribly. You need to gather the data about how your content is being perceived, and make your own critical evaluation. Could you have done things better? What did you do particularly well? Is this lining up with your brand identity which you outlined in your unique selling points? Evaluating your work like this over time helps you to mould your brand into the one you envisioned.

After a while, this obviously gets a little monotonous. That's why I said earlier that, to succeed, you have to enjoy the process. Sometimes I get overwhelmed with the endless cycle of content generation because, as soon as one piece of filming is done, there is no reward, break or pat on the back. You simply move on to the next one. There is no end goal, only an endless forward momentum. Thankfully I enjoy the process, so while it can be overwhelming at times, it's mostly exciting.

Obviously all of this sounds like a lot of work, or at least like a lot more work than you might have imagined some social media superstars doing. The harsh truth is that many of these people do absolutely nothing. Plenty are lazy and have simply attracted fame based on luck of the draw or the genetic lottery. If you're not one of these people then you're probably going to have to work for it.

However, even those who work for it (or not) can and do fail. I see successful people in the industry failing all of the time, and because a lot of preventable reasons such as complacency or entitlement causing a disruption to the system. For example, a successful creator might experience a shift in their values over time and no longer be the person they once were (incongruity with step 1). They might reduce their efforts in creating (flouting step 2) because they've already 'made it'. They might no longer add value to their community and eventually suffer for it. Or maybe they failed to adapt (step 3) and their content stagnated. They might try to recycle what worked before, without realising that it no longer resonates. Whether you have found success or not, to maintain a position in the market you have to constantly adapt and evaluate.

The same principles apply to brands. In a more traditional marketing sense, they have been doing this for a long time. Brands position themselves among competitors, identify their USPs and competitive advantage. They then tailor their marketing messages to align with these ideas. Social media is marketing. Brands must create content with the goal of outlining their brand identity and creating a community.

Let's look at the social media giant Gymshark, for example. Gymshark uses popular fitness influencers to represent them as an elite brand of gym clothing. Their earlier brand identity online was admirable and motivational, as if holding an elusive god-like status in fitness. As the brand grew, they evolved to develop more of an entertaining, inclusive, personable identity to accommodate a larger community of people. They post funnier content that is far less serious.

What if creating content for a clothing company differs in some way to other companies? Okay, let's look at a brand that sells ... water pistols (the first random thing to pop in my head). They could take a boring approach to marketing in every piece of content, without regard for the community they wish to create or their niche position. They could create content demonstrating that their pistols work and they're cheaper than the next alternative, which would be dull and unlikely to be shared. Or they could decide to be a less serious brand that represents fun for adults and children alike and adjust their content to viral trends, with images of wet family members and friends spraying each other with their water pistols. The content would be more shareable and would convey values of playfulness and fun that further cement their brand identity.

People respond to feelings and values rather than products or services. This can be utilised by any brand offering a product or a service in the market and just requires some brainstorming and abstract thinking.

If you're reading this and you are wanting to start a social media presence for yourself or your company, I strongly suggest you just make a start. There will be no perfect time and the more you practise the aforementioned steps, the better you will become at them and the more you will learn. Start now and your future self will thank you!

Oh, and if you're a water pistol company wanting to steal my idea, don't even think about it as I have already patented it and will sue you for billions.

# 29

# Why you need to welcome the haters

I first started a fitness Instagram in 2013. I used a pseudonym out of fear the people who knew me would find out about my gym photos. Looking back on it now is quite funny, but I clearly had anxiety about what others would think of me and it felt real!

I had an irrational fear of receiving hate and so I began posting from the perspective of a cocky, confident guy to mask my insecurities. As a result, I was met with even *more* hate than I'd originally feared. Without realising it, my overconfident facade had basically signalled to the internet, 'Hey guys, I think I'm awesome. I'm better than you, time to take me down a peg – let's go!' I lasted a month before realising it was a horrible idea and I should start again on my personal account. So one day I built up the courage to post a photo of my flexed lats in the gym to my 757 followers. I wasn't acting cocky this time, but I was ready to deal with the hate once again.

To my surprise, there was no hate. Not even one comment. I slowly continued posting and two years later I had accumulated around 5000 followers who were very much used to my typical gym photos. I thought I had finally overcome my fear of hate. But that was only because I was yet to truly receive any. In my mind, I figured that as long as I was genuinely being myself and not projecting my insecurities in the form of false confidence, I would be safe.

That has been right for the most part. However, like anything, there is always a minority. I mean, there is a minority of people that believe that the moon landing isn't real, Bill Gates created fake snow and if they move one step too far they'll fall off the edge of the Earth. Among the flat-Earthers and Moon-landing deniers, there exists a minority of people who are going to find something or someone to hate on no matter what.

They might be so dissatisfied with their own life that they need to project that negativity onto others to comfort themselves. They might be jealous or angry, or maybe they've been robbed once by someone who looks like you. You cannot know what someone else is going through or has dealt with in the past. So when I see haters doing this now, I try to approach the situation with empathy and openness.

I really try not to take it personally (even though some people are gifted in the art of piercing my deepest insecurities), and for the most part I can remain unfazed. How? Well, because I know that whoever is trying to bring me down is clearly suffering in some kind of way. They have to be! If they weren't suffering, then they'd be far too content with their own lives to rage about anything trivial I may or may not have done. This is what I tell young guys and girls who ask me how I 'deal with haters'. I also tell them not to give people unnecessary reason to hate them (such as adopting a fake persona), and to try to put themselves in the hater's shoes and feel sorry for them if possible. Empathy is a great way to shift the social hierarchy that you create in your mind.

However, no empathetic mental gymnastics could have prepared 20-year-old me for the most hate I'd ever received in my life … All because of a dirty mirror.

Social media personalities go through phases. One day an account is popular for providing quality information and the next day another one is popular for 'calling people out' and creating drama.

In 2015, the trend at the time on one popular account was to call fitness bodies out for Photoshopping their physiques. It was the golden era of Photoshop and a time when most people would be fooled by pinched tums, enlarged bums, bulging biceps and 3D triceps. This account would post other people's photos and his follower army would expose them as frauds, doling out punishment usually taking the form of immediate mass amounts of hate on the infringer's profile so that the person, their friends, their neighbours and their mums would know what a filthy, lying Photoshopping sack of shit they were.

This was before the days of Instagram comment moderation and violations of community guidelines, so it's safe to say it was not a very safe place for those who dabbled in the dark arts of photo manipulation. But, just like in every other penal system before it, there lies the danger of punishing the innocent. You guessed it: I ended up campaigning for my innocence amidst a barrage of hatred.

The photo in question was a mirror selfie I took at a gym when I was at my leanest. Thanks to my genetics, my lats insert quite low and my waist shrinks when I'm lean, so with a little angulation and torso rotation, I could present the illusion of a V taper. A real statue of David (Copperfield perhaps).

Sadly, the gym staff skipped their weekly bathroom clean as often as I skipped leg day, with the result of a filthy mirror covered in vertical streaks and splashes. To the untrained eye, these vertical streaks almost looked like tiles behind me. I say 'almost', because the streaks weren't uniform. One happened to draw a line in precisely the same angle as my waist. It genuinely looked like I had taken a photo, shrunk my waist digitally and accidentally warped the tiles behind me in the process. But, as you know, there *were* no tiles behind me. It was an illusion!

To the army of Photoshop hunters, this photo was a crime of the highest order. I screenshotted the comments as my life unfolded before me, and for the first time I felt genuinely anxious about the hate I was getting. Like all of my hard work was now ruined and the reputation I had worked so hard to build was lost forever.

Looking back at their comments now, I just laugh. Mark said, 'Your gains bend walls bruh.' Nice and simple! Charles was having a bad day as he wrote, 'Nice Photoshopping you fucking piece of shit scumbag c\*\*t.' That one now makes me smile. And finally, Austin wins the day as he so eloquently gathers his thoughts and calls me, 'The Wall Bending C\*\*t.' It's a title that sounds so cool I wish I deserved it, like a superpower that mere mortals wish to have but could never control.

Long story short, I ended up messaging the account and he acknowledged the streaks, apologised for his judgement and deleted the post from his page. I recovered from my initial anxiety.

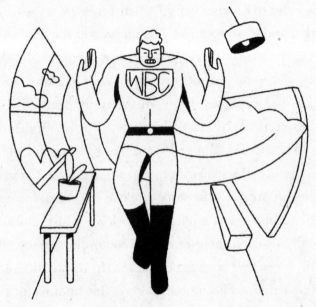

Haters exist, but the truth of the matter is: if you don't have haters, you're not doing anything worthwhile. Haters are a sign that what you're doing is powerful enough to make people feel something (on both ends of the spectrum). They're a sign that your actions are provoking jealousy or shaking belief systems. So, instead of fearing online hatred, *welcome* the haters. Invite them in, sit them down and make them a cup of freshly brewed hater tea.

Trust me, the opposite of receiving hate isn't love and endless support. The opposite is being so plain, neutral and vanilla that nobody cares about you or what you're doing. Do something worthwhile, that is bold enough to make people support you on one end, and make a few miserable people try and take you down a notch on the other. Now I am free to be as much of a wall-bending C as I like.

# 30

# How to improve your confidence and harness motivation

My first 'sit down' YouTube video began in my room and ended in a wave of anxiety. I set my camera up on a tripod and started *trying* to speak about the topic I'd set myself. I emphasise the word 'trying' because I turned off the camera after what felt like hours of awkward silence between episodes of senseless rambling. Filming was very new to me and the act of talking to the camera or large groups made me extremely nervous. In fact, when preparing group presentations at university, I would take charge of the team (portraying a false sense of confidence) and delegate tasks so I could relieve myself of the duty of presenting. Public speaking was a nightmare for me and filming that first video gave me similar feelings. To this day it remains the only video I have filmed and never posted. Maybe I could post it if

I title it 'MILEY CYRUS LOOKALIKE FREEZES FOR 24 HOURS'.

I remember coming very close to putting the camera down and forgetting about YouTube altogether after that. I felt like I didn't have what it took, I had no confidence, I sucked, my face was red, no one was going to help me get better, everyone was going to laugh at my red face, why was my face so red? For some reason – against the kind advice of my aforementioned inner thoughts – I slept on it and tried again the next day.

Years later I'd be speaking at events in front of hundreds of people with ease, and filming videos for millions with sincere confidence. The change didn't happen overnight and, contrary to what I had believed, faking confidence isn't fooling (or helping) anyone, especially myself.

Entering my early 20s with a low level of confidence was not part of the game plan.

I listened to a lot of self-help podcasts in an attempt to work on the issue. Interestingly, nearly everything I read or listened to told me to manifest confidence through daily affirmations, claiming that eventually I'd embody that confidence. I know it sounds a little bit corny, or silly, or maybe like the dumbest shitty advice one could ever receive. That's because it is. At the time, though, I needed all the help I could get. I found myself in my car in the mornings repeating the affirmation, 'I am confident and I am motivated.' In hindsight that was about as useful as me saying, 'I will win the lottery today.'

Am I confident now, years later? Yes. Was it due to this method of confidence boosting? No, not really. I discovered something about confidence almost by accident. Well, two things really. One: confidence and motivation are highly linked. Two: they are linked through success. The more small successes (or wins) you have in any given field, the more confident you are within yourself and the more motivation you have. No matter how hard I tried to portray confidence on camera in my first video, I literally could not do it. In the battle of Anxiety vs False Confidence, Anxiety almost always wins. No matter how much you puff your chest out and put on a show, your trembling, sweaty hands and shaky voice will prove that physiology is tough to control through sheer will.

Furthermore, if you have no confidence, the voice in your head will always be there telling you, 'You can't do this,' despite any efforts to silence it.

So instead of trying to fake anything, I just focused on the small task at hand: my next video. If you zoom out and take a wider view of what I did over time, I practised filming more, I liked working the camera and learned how to make videos more enjoyable to watch.

Slowly, slowly I gained confidence through posting hundreds of videos online, each trying to be better than the last and therefore each acting as a small win I could add to my internal list of successes. I didn't try to be 'the confident guy' after a 10-second affirmation, I gave it time and let myself truly become that person through a natural process. I essentially did this by accident.

After a few hundred YouTube videos, the fear that I once had was non-existent. I proved to myself that I *could* do it. It's as simple as that.

Confidence in any particular area is the belief that you can do something that pertains to that area or field. The only way to grow it is to push your comfort zone and do more. Motivation is similar in this sense, as most people view motivation as the spark that gets you going, the fleeting urge to drag your body into action or the pure physiological energy that drives your every move. But what a lot of people forget is that motivation requires action first.

Let's say you want to start working towards a new goal – maybe joining a gym and committing to workouts. Perhaps you watched a Goggins video that triggered a mental shift and sparked the first move (this is most people's definition of motivation). But sadly, that initial change in mentality doesn't last too long and the brain has a very persuasive way of convincing you that you no longer need or want that goal. Eventually the mindset fizzles along with the dream.

If that kind of motivation doesn't work, what does? Winning does. The *only* way to continue that motivation is to give yourself frequent successes or wins.

Using the example of going to the gym, these wins can be as simple as just turning up or achieving a personal best in a given set. The win will trigger a dopamine release and contribute to your sense of drive and pursuit. So to defy the status quo, you don't actually need motivation before the success. You need successes for motivation.

As cryptic as that sounds, it's true. There is nothing more motivating at a psychological level than witnessing yourself making progress. Don't forget, in the beginning the act of getting out of the house and turning up is progress.

After a while, motivation changes. It turns into behaviours that form a part of your identity and you no longer even have to think about them, or it transfers to another task or desire you wish to accomplish. This is why people like to credit their success to discipline as opposed to motivation. You know the saying: 'Motivation gets you started, discipline keeps you going.' Don't even get me started. Without outlining the differences between discipline and motivation, it's merely a cool-sounding phrase. It's as helpful as saying about financial success, 'The Poor lack money. The Rich do not.' Imagine if your financial adviser said that to you after assessing your situation. You'd probably murder him, and then be told by your lawyer that, 'Innocent people do not murder.' Discipline just means the person has made their goals a part of their lifestyle and – eventually identity – through the process of small successes and perseverance.

If going to the gym has become part of your identity, it's far easier to train on the days you don't feel like it than when you're just starting out and wondering if all this gym stuff is really worth it.

So confidence and motivation are two sides of the same coin, and they both require action to set them in motion. However, I found that confidence was multifaceted. On one hand, my own confidence increased by becoming more proficient, but on the other hand, confidence is closely tied to long held beliefs that we all have about ourselves and carry with us. I became confident in front of a camera in my early 20s, but that didn't necessarily make me a truly confident person.

I wasn't fully able to be myself and express who I was without fear of judgement. If I wanted to talk to a girl, I would feel like I had no confidence at all due to these hardwired beliefs that I wasn't good enough (which probably stemmed from my low self-esteem and insecurities in high school). So even though I became proficient and confident in one area, I still had to consciously let go of the limiting beliefs I'd been carrying for so long that were holding me back.

Every failed conversation or embarrassing confrontation would be embedded subconsciously in my mind and would dissuade me from approaching 'that girl' and being myself. It's like the brain keeps an internal tally of events that confirm these undermining beliefs. I remember literally analysing (through journalling) what my fears were and, to my surprise, they were completely silly. *What's the worst-case scenario if I approach an attractive girl and start a conversation? Um, maybe there will be an awkward silence and she'll cut my legs off.* No, probably not.

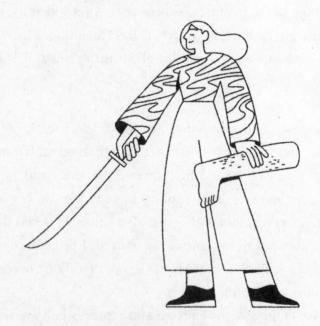

I realised my fear was actually that a particular failure might worsen my already dwindling confidence. So I had to do three things. Firstly, I let go of damaging long-held destructive beliefs about myself (you aren't good with girls, you don't deserve good things etc). Secondly, I changed my relationship with failure. I started to look at failure as a positive chance to learn. If I failed, I'd still reward myself for trying and then look for the silver lining as a lesson to be learned. If I approached a girl, whether I had a good conversation or a terrible one, I'd still give myself credit for doing it. If I volunteered for a public speaking event, I wouldn't base my success on my performance but would base it on simply turning up. Then, as turning up became easier I would slowly raise the bar. The goal then shifted to delivering the best version of myself possible.

The final task for bullet-proofing confidence came from repetition. You have to convince yourself wholeheartedly that you are the type of person who deserves confidence. You cannot trick yourself into believing it, because you are smart and will see through your own bullshit no matter how many times you yell it in the mirror. Repetition will get you better at whatever it is that you're doing. In time it will stack up to prove you are who you say you are.

In one of my YouTube videos on developing confidence I received a message from a young guy named Josh. He told me he had no confidence or self-esteem and his dream was to improve, but he didn't know where to begin. After chatting further, he admitted that his goal was to enter the fitness industry and spread messages about health and fitness, but he was terrified to publicly post his opinions because he felt like he didn't know enough. Instead of telling him to fake it and just *be* confident, I said that his hesitations were perfectly normal. I told him to learn more about fitness and improve his competency, and then he would feel confident and entitled to share his opinions.

His next step was letting go of his fear of judgement. He was worried about receiving hate online for posting fitness content, and so I told him about when I first started.

I started fitness content under the pseudonym @young_zyzz. Cringe, I know. But Zyzz was one of my adolescent fitness idols. He was the epitome of confidence, so I adopted a false bravado and conveyed pure cockiness in my photos. I'd post a physique photo with a caption to the effect of 'Everyone is admiring me. Are you jealous?' As I have already admitted, I was met with my deepest fear: hate.

Wow, I was receiving hate after telling everyone how good I was and that they should be jealous? Makes sense actually. As you know if you've stayed the course and read the chapters in order, I deleted the account immediately and built the courage to post on my own account. This time there would be no alter ego and I would just be unequivocally me. Not because I'd reached any profound realisation about the beauty of authenticity, but because the other plan sure as hell did not work. The result: very little to no hate. People love to find enormous egos and knock them down a peg, but only assholes tear down people who are being genuine and authentic.

In my history of social media I have received little hate. Not none of course, as we share this world with some of the strangest, most psychopathic, bitter and miserable people, who would hate on a charity worker for their haircut. But when I was being myself and expressing who I was, no opinion from someone else could really change how I felt. This took more confidence than I ever had previously.

*

True confidence runs deep and is up to the individual to address and work on. For me, it was about becoming competent enough to feel like I knew what I was doing and then work on the beliefs holding me back from being my true self.

I, like many others, also suffered from an identity issue. After years of telling myself I wasn't confident, it was truly difficult to shake that idea and *feel* confident, even with competence or acquired skills. Some of us have to consciously work on identifying as a person with confidence, until it becomes firmly entrenched in who you are. I genuinely believe this is a malleable trait, because I have experienced it first-hand.

I used to imagine a hypothetical version of myself who acted with confidence and then tried to act in accordance with how that confident Zac would act. What I found was that it was quite easy to be confident with practice and the right mentality. Motivation was essentially my desire made into a game plan. Both had to be worked on for long enough until they were forged into my identity. So I wasn't just the same person with an extra boost of self-esteem; I became a new person. I went from 'the fat kid' to 'the fitness guy'. I went from terrified Miley Cyrus to a confident public speaker.

The sad truth is that sometimes these stories can be harmful, but the up-side lies in the fact that these stories are ever changing and can empower us to be more than what we could imagine. We can in fact be the author of our own story, but it doesn't come easy and it does requires action. Don't wait for a miracle, don't wait to get a PhD to talk about your passion and don't wait for the right *time* to take action. Don't think. Just go, now, because it will trigger a cascade of behaviours and events that will one day forge you into the person you want to be.

In other words, young Miley, staring in painfully awkward silence at the camera, didn't have to do anything else but show up, learn from his mistakes and give it time. Eventually he'd become the person he aspired to be. Wait, so does that make me Hannah Montana? Dammit, I'd like a redo on the analogy please. It's already been edited? Shit.

# 31

# The Harry Potter Method

To this day, I still get called Harry Spotter. I've even met people in the industry who scream in delight, 'YOU'RE HARRY SPOTTER?' after finally putting the pieces together. I can trace this back to when I was eight years old and Harry Potter was my favourite dress-up character. Somehow each birthday and Christmas, a wand and a magic kit would make it onto my presents list. One day, I did my best Harry Potter impression to an audience of three: Joel, Mum and Dad. Solid response. I repeated the performance 12 years later to an audience of several hundred million. Just a slightly bigger audience.

But I didn't create my first viral video as a means of going viral, I did it for the same reason as I dressed up the first time ... fun.

By 2015, my social media following had picked up and I'd reached around 30,000 followers on Instagram through posting content of my physique and everything fitness. I remember being messaged by a man named Andrew who was the owner of fitness apparel brand Strong Liftwear. He asked if I was available to do a photoshoot for his brand.

I could barely hold my phone. I was shaking with excitement and could not believe the opportunity. Ever since I started getting into the social media side of fitness, I had aspired to be a part of two brands only: Strong Liftwear (SLW) and Gymshark. SLW was very popular in Australia and Gymshark was becoming a world-renowned fitness brand. Now I was actually talking to the owner of one of them. He told me we would shoot as soon as he returned from his holiday in a couple of weeks. I responded with a fervent yes and hoped with every ounce of my being that he wouldn't change his mind in that time. (I was sure he would figure out he'd made a mistake and proceed to ignore me thereafter.)

To my surprise, things were in fact too good AND true, so I did my first photoshoot in his home studio and then in an abandoned warehouse (spoiler: I didn't get murdered). He spoke of potential future sponsorship. As a 20-year-old wanting to take a firm step deeper into the industry, I couldn't have been more excited. Shortly after, he was once again true to his word and he signed me on as an athlete with a discount code and everything! Life made.

In my time working with the brand, Andrew took me under his wing. He was in his early 30s and had quit his job in financial recruitment to start his own apparel business. Clearly it worked out and he had left his day job to pursue a life of entrepreneurship. I had absolutely no idea what he saw in me and I was constantly perplexed, but I didn't want to question his judgement. Somehow me saying, 'I think you've made a grave mistake in investing in me,' wouldn't work out for either of us, so I kept it to myself.

Andrew then guided me in the right direction for furthering my career in social media. He encouraged me to start a YouTube channel. When I say forced, I don't mean with a gun to the head, 'Film this video or I will literally shoot you on camera for the world to see.' He encouraged me to start showing my personality, as he clearly saw something I didn't, and for that I'll always be extremely grateful. So I listened to Andrew and whatever he said soon became advice I took seriously.

I began posting fitness videos and continued my regular fitness content on Instagram. This was the time before the artificially intelligent complexities of deep fakes. Face swap apps were just emerging and I then took advantage of the new technology. I've always had a love for impersonations, constantly doing accents and voices of celebrities. I had a knack for some but others were too shocking to be heard outside of the confines of my own car, so I was sure to play to my strengths.

This one particular app sparked my interest because it was the most impressive, realistic Harry Potter face swapping tech I had ever seen. For weeks I recorded random videos acting as the young wizard and sent them to my friends. I filled my camera roll with what I thought to be hilarious videos, and among them was one I sent to Andrew. I was wearing SLW and said to the camera in my best Harry Potter impression, 'Check out the newest Hogwarts school uniform … Hagrid check it out. I'm fuckin' massive mate.' Andrew replied laughing, saying, 'You HAVE to post that.' I told him no way in hell, it was for his eyes only, and he replied with, 'Trust me, it's hilarious. Post it.'

So, as usual, I listened. I filmed a few extra bits to add to it, and then posted it on my Facebook page with the simple caption: 'If Harry Potter was a bodybuilder.'

Seeing it reach 20,000 views in one morning freaked me out! I was already ecstatic. Over the ensuing weeks, it had gone completely viral and was shared by every major Facebook group at the time, including the pages of big names like 50 Cent. It was a weird feeling at the time, having millions of people watch me just joking around. And it was a huge stretch away from my usual fitness content.

I had no idea how or why the only thing that went viral and threw me a taste of superficial internet fame was something completely unrelated to how I looked. I thought that it was *all* about looks and people succeeded based on appearance. In hindsight, it's clear now that the only reason it did work was because it wasn't superficial. It was something original that came out of my brain that I found funny but had been too scared to show people. I don't even know what I was afraid of when I think about it, but it must've been some fear of judgement. 'What if people think it's not funny? What if it flops?' Questions that I never should've been posing in the first place.

Most people live with a debilitating fear of being judged … a fear of what others might think. I don't use the word 'debilitating' lightly here. This particular fear crushes self-esteem and extinguishes any trace of potential. It tells you you're not special and that the world will punish you for trying. It's arguably the most dangerous fear due to its ability to keep you prisoner to a world of boring comfort and ordinariness.

Ironically, the fear of not being special enough to pursue something actually makes you less special. It makes you do less and fear more. I couldn't see it at the time, but my biggest strength was not my slightly above average physique but my quirks and personality. That's what sets me apart, that's what I need to pursue and that's what Fluffy is guarding on the third floor. Sorry, I had to include a Harry Potter reference.

As I have said before, it took me a long time to learn to embrace my peculiarities, because I was scared of what other people would think. Some people are afraid to try something new, to pursue their interests, to put themselves out there, because of that same fear. Without sounding like a preachy therapist, this fear actually gives you even more reason to do what you're scared of. Because once you are out there and you realise that your fears were irrational, you'll be far more equipped to do more with yourself and see what you're capable of.

It won't always be obvious fears that hold you back, however. Some of you might put yourself out there and your fear could very well come true. Let's say you're like me and deep down you want to post a video of something you found funny in the hope that others might share in the humour, but you're scared you will receive hate. I'm not going to tell you that your fear is irrational and people won't hate on you. You might post it and read the very comments you feared. In fact, at some point you definitely will.

There is a silver lining in this, though, because that very exercise will teach you that even though you might be hilarious you cannot and will not always please everyone. Furthermore, the more important lesson lies in not deriving value from random people's opinions. So instead of avoiding your fear you just developed a way to overcome it and set yourself one step further towards your own potential.

I genuinely think posting that video was a turning point in my life and I wouldn't even have a career if it wasn't for that. Not for the numbers or being known as the Harry Spotter guy, but for teaching me that what sets you apart from others is not a dull conformity to what everyone else is doing. As I have said before, what sets you apart and makes you different can't be distilled perfectly in one sentence. If I were to try (and let's take a stab) I would say that what makes you unique is a rich tapestry of personal experience, personality traits, interests, fascinations and physical attributes. No one really told me this back then. I had to figure out what made me different through doing what I believed to be fun and completely disregarding what other people thought.

As a kid, this meant dressing up as Harry and casting spells. As an adult this meant dressing up as Harry, flexing my bicep and telling the world that 'I'm fucking massive'.

# 32

# The difference between opportunity and danger

Looking back, it seems that being an online fitness persona in 2015 was still relatively new and highly esteemed in the fitness industry. If you went to the gym daily, you knew who the few fitness personalities were. They were kind of like low-level B-list celebrities: inaccessible and mysterious. Nowadays everyone knows someone who is some kind of fitness influencer, but back when I was just stepping foot into this world there were a lot of mysteries that I simply accepted. Such as how someone can have so many abs, what magical powers creatine monohydrate actually possesses and what the fuck is with all of these weird old guys messaging me?

As a sheltered 20-year-old I was very trusting. If someone told me something, I took their word for it. If they promised me something, I believed them because why wouldn't I? In my blissfully ignorant mind, people didn't have hidden agendas

239

or malevolent egos. I believed the world wanted to help me because it said it did. So when I started to receive messages from a much older man (let's call him Elmer) telling me he was going to make me the 'next best thing', just like I'd done with other successful influencers Albert and Ernest, of course I believed him. (I obviously can't name names here so please excuse my pseudonyms.)

Elmer started off by complimenting my physique, and I was genuinely appreciative. My ego hadn't experienced much flattery so I was receptive to it. He then started throwing things out there like, 'I could turn you into a champion if you trained with me, just like I did with Bert,' and 'Trust me, if you come to the States and train with me I'll have you looking like Ernie.' It went on and on.

Just to paint the picture for you, this man didn't exactly look like a personal trainer. He didn't look like he'd actually seen a personal trainer in his life. Skinny, flabby and about to cark it if he took the wrong step.

At the time I took it all at face value and found his approaches enticing. He seems credible, right? He's name-dropping these other young guys, he must be legit? I actually began to plan my US trip but had to postpone due to having only a few dollars to my name – my job working the local pharmacy's cash register wasn't so lucrative. Shoutout to the pharmacy for potentially saving my ass in the most literal sense.

If I received those messages at this point in my life my first thoughts would be: 1) What does this guy *actually* want? (Probably money or something weirder). And 2) What does this guy have on these other young guys? (Probably money, access to illicit substances, unethical contracts or some other form of leverage.)

I would then proceed to ignore this weirdo because I know that the world will overpromise and underdeliver again and again. Not because the world is evil and people are out to get you, but because people are self-serving animals and fallible in nature.

Back then I had not experienced being truly let down before. I was yet to experience of business deals that fell through, people breaking their word and simple blind optimism in schemes that would just never eventuate. I remember thinking, 'Wow this guy is so kind, he wants me to be famous. I want to be famous. Well we both want the same thing, so let's do it.' I didn't even think for a second that maybe he was just deluded.

Don't get me wrong, there are definitely people out there that genuinely see something in another person and want the best for them, but if there's a situation where someone is coming on very strong in their seeming support, it's important to protect yourself with the assumption that they are in it for themselves and themselves only. Some people see an opportunity to exploit others for their own gain and they will take advantage of other people's ignorance.

The weirdest thing about it all is the number of weird old guys in the fitness space that do the same thing. It's like an industry full of innocent young sculpted bodies somehow attracts creepy old men. Strange.

Thankfully, after telling Elmer that I wouldn't be making the trip after all, he continued to incessantly harass my inbox. Thankfully common sense then prevailed and I realised that this guy was just plain weird. Blocked.

Luckily for me that was the worst of it as far as weird old men go. But not disappointment in general – I still had many lessons to learn.

I was contacted one year later by a marketing company with huge plans to scale up my online coaching business. I was at uni at the time and writing PDF training programs for people, leveraging my slowly growing platform to get a handful of clients to write plans for. I would get up at 5am on weekends to write programs – and I loved it! I even saved up enough money to quit my part-time job selling supplements at ASN to finally work for myself. I had saved up around $20,000 in total when I first received an offer from a marketing company.

Back then I had never heard the word 'scale' outside of the context of a gym bathroom. Their idea was to scale up my company through running Facebook ads to generate new clients and make more money for me and a nice little slice for themselves. I met these guys and liked them. They seemed nice and like they genuinely believed in me. They even showed me the forecasted projections which indicated that with just $30,000 of ad spend, I would be on track to generate over a million dollars in revenue.

They were shocked by the projections and so was I. I knew that these guys weren't scammers because they were yet to even profit from my money so I had to believe them!

I know what you're thinking. 'Come on, Zac, where did they get the figures from? What assumptions were made in the process? Surely you didn't jump straight in?' You probably know where this is going, I've set it up nicely. I jumped so far in, head-first, straight into the shallow end.

I paid my entire savings up front and even convinced my parents to chip in and pay the remaining budget. Taking out Facebook ads was a new idea for all of us and I told Mum and Dad that they couldn't argue with the figures, so they should just trust me. Did I generate the projected $180,000 in my first month? Absolutely fucking not. I turned over a few hundred bucks and the results were so bad that the company apologised, said they didn't know what happened and refused to take any additional payment for the service.

Now that I think about it, it's a pretty interesting service. 'Give me your life savings and I'll burn it for a small fee.'

I honestly didn't blame the company. They genuinely believed it would work. Their assumptions were way off and they were obviously out of their depth in the context of fitness, but they weren't out to get me; they just didn't know any better. It was at that point of losing my life savings, and most importantly letting my parents down, that I learned the valuable lesson that Elmer tried to teach me a year earlier: don't rely on someone else to make it happen for you.

In hindsight, I should've done the research. I should've been self-educated on paid marketing before thinking that this one leap would make all the difference. I also should've thought about the simple fact that people are not selfless angels. They overpromise and underdeliver every single day and it's up to us to use our own knowledge to separate opportunity from danger and a good decision from a bad one.

So if someone ever tells you something that's too good to be true, don't take it at face value, and whatever you do: do not catch a plane to an old weirdo's house just to realise that you flew halfway around the world to visit an old weirdo in his house.

# 33
# How to make money from social media

I was around 21 when I built up the courage to tell my friends and family that I wanted to pursue a career in social media. Everyone's immediate reaction was to look at me, puzzled, as if I'd told them I wanted to follow my passion in teaching monkeys how to juggle. Then, still as if I showed them a video of me with a chimp holding juggling balls, they would ask me in a very concerned manner, 'That's great but can you make money from it?'

To be honest, I hadn't yet thought that far ahead. I told them that I'd figure it out. I didn't even know if there was much money, if any, to be made in social media, I just knew it was what I wanted to do. However, for many years I'd kept that dream to myself out of fear of being treated like a failed circus trainer.

For some reason I just decided to start telling people my goals and owning them. Perhaps I was looking for some accountability, or maybe I wanted to convince myself that this was happening. Either way, I am very happy that I put my intentions out into the world (mainly for myself to hear).

Note that this was the early days of social media, so I can't entirely blame the older generation for their monetary concerns. However, I still get the exact same questions now when I tell people what I do for a living. Some of them assume I make no income at all, while most assume I do it all for some free poached eggs at the local cafe. But now, instead of responding with a half-hearted answer of, 'I'll figure it out,' I can barely hide my grin as I say, 'You have *no* idea.'

Social media allows people to influence other people's behaviour. The more eyes you have on you, the more people you can potentially influence. This was common sense to me in the early days; I could see it was just like how movie stars and celebrities had influence over the general population. I thought that if I couldn't make money directly through companies on social media, I could make it indirectly through boosting my presence in the space and creating a genuine trust between myself and my audience – to be an influencer.

I started out immediately replying to all comments and was grateful for the support I received. I think that this was a major factor in my ability to create a community, as everyone felt valued and respected. I knew back then that I could monetise my following somehow, but I wasn't ready to and I didn't have the means.

Today the possibilities to monetise one's social media through an array of avenues, such as offering exclusive content, brand deals, direct monetisation, or marketing one's own separate business, is just about endless. I'm going to be completely transparent here and share with you things I've never told anyone to give you an accurate insight into the job from my perspective. Let's go through each of these briefly.

## Offering exclusive content

Since social media was flooded with free content (before 2016 by my estimate), companies saw the opportunity to monetise exclusive content to those willing to pay to see more from their favourite creator. Take OnlyFans for example. This was founded in 2016 by British businessman Tim Stockley, alongside his brother and father. The site enables users/performers to directly monetise content by posting their exclusive content to those who pay a given fee. This allowed adult entertainers and social media personalities worldwide to directly monetise content without being banned or flagged by Instagram's community guidelines.

The market was huge. In 2021, the company reported earnings of US$932 million and creators earned nearly $4 billion. While adult entertainers thrived on the platform, many social media influencers would use it just to post photos they might normally post on Instagram, only there it would be monetised. I personally know people earning five figures every month on this site, making it a very tempting experience.

I remember telling my dad about OnlyFans. I was telling him how much money these guys were making on this platform, with zero intention of doing so myself but just as a point of interest. Instead of shaking his head in disappointment, Dad looked at me and said, 'You've GOTTA do it, son!' I then said, 'Dad, I don't want to post my nudes online,' in the same way

I would tell Dad that I didn't want to take the bins out. I'm fairly certain I'm still the only person on Earth that has uttered such a phrase. He said, 'No, you don't post nudes, just post the photos you normally post on your Instagram, like undies pics, and make thousands off whoever wants to pay!' The man had a point; he is an opportunist and a businessman after all.

But knowing what I know about brand image and association, I politely declined my dad's suggestion.

OnlyFans aside, there are other ways to monetise exclusive content, as many businesses have created family-friendly platforms for creators to post additional content. YouTube created subscription services to compete with other online subscription services that host creators and their content. I have never jumped over to this, as I could barely create enough content anyway. If I did any extra, it would probably come at the expense of free content for others. So I have left this avenue relatively unexplored.

## Brand deals

My first brand deal was an Instagram post for a teeth-whitening company for $1000 when I hit 100,000 Instagram followers. I thought I had absolutely made it. In 2022, I signed a brand deal to showcase a new laptop for well into five figures for a couple of Instagram posts, stories and YouTube videos. The amount of money in endorsements is unreal. Those with smaller followings will often accept a simple complimentary breakfast in exchange for their posting, yet I'd much rather pay my way like anyone else and save the paid content creation for those that align with my values … and who pay to have me showcase it.

With that said, it can't always be about the money. Since I started, I've only ever accepted brand deals with companies that I actually see value in.

I would lose trust in my audience if they tried something I'd promoted and were disappointed. For example, I've worked with hair-product companies like BluMaan, clothing companies like Cuts and Legend London, supplement companies like EHPlabs and gym wear brands like Gymshark. All of these brands I have actually made personal purchases with, so it is a complete no-brainer to partner with them and promote the products on my platform. It's not a good long-term strategy to take on as much as you can get regardless of what it is. You permanently damage your own reputation (and ability to cash in later) when your audience sees you as a sell-out.

Nevertheless, I've always tried to give my own personal spin on my sponsored content to make it more entertaining and less 'salesy' to my audience, even if it was to my detriment. One time I secured a deal with an audiobook company. I proceeded to dress up as a blind man and promote audiobooks as I cooked dinner (I put my dog in the oven), pet my dog (I pet a roast chicken) and even while driving (I crashed). While they said it *was* funny, it was not appropriate for an ad and they kindly requested that I remove it. Oh well, I had to try! In hindsight, this skit isn't appropriate in any scenario, but often my attempts at humour override everything else.

### Direct monetisation

YouTube and Facebook now offer direct payment via ad revenue. In simple terms, companies pay YouTube to host their ads. Viewers watch the ads on your videos and you get a small kickback. The more viewers watching the ad, the larger the kickback. YouTube doesn't have a set dollar per views that they'll pay, as the exact number is influenced by many factors such as the niche you're in and who your viewers are. For example, someone who posts entrepreneurial videos will receive more money per thousand views (CPM) than someone who posts gaming videos, because the audience of the former is likely to have more disposable income and higher spending habits.

In my case, I have an older audience on YouTube compared to those playing to gaming channels with young teenagers, so my CPM is relatively high. That said, to give you a rough idea, when I was posting one or two videos a week, each getting one to two hundred thousand views, I would receive around US$5000–$7000 per month. Compare that to some of my friends in the industry: when they would get around a million views per video, posting twice weekly, they would receive around US$80,000 per month. Absolutely crazy money for doing something that's so fun.

There are so many other avenues for social media monetisation. To name a few more, Twitch has a similar way that users can monetise their gaming – users can take a portion of the revenue generated byads. Twitch creators can also make money via subscriptions from those who pay a monthly fee to watch them stream, as well as one-off donations. I even know people making six figures a month from posting Snapchat stories alone – so you have a lot of options!

YouTube is tempting for the monetisation appeal, but just like anything that uses money as a draw card, it's also dangerous. It can make you create content for what the system prefers, not what you *want* to do.

I always wanted to make videos to help people have better lives. Whether that was directly, through fitness, health and lifestyle advice, or indirectly, through providing laughs and good vibes, that's my underlying motivation. I never wanted to become a a sell-out that creates videos for money, as that would change the purpose for me and I would no longer love it. Who knows, maybe I would love the six-figure months, but either way, there is a careful path to tread if you want to succeed in creating videos favoured by the algorithm while also being true to your purpose.

I haven't quite nailed it yet, but those who succeed in both absolutely crush the game. Many of my 'work mates' in the fitness industry do this and it's inspiring to see!

## Marketing an additional business

This is what I primarily use my platform for, as I have been able to promote my online coaching program to help as many people as possible on a larger scale. I built up this business and then branched out into something entirely different when creating the pyjama brand Slouch Potato with my brother (see more in chapter 35).

Using your social media platform to build up your own business is a method of diversification in creating something larger than yourself. I always wanted to branch out into a different field and create something bigger than my name and encompassing more of a movement of individuals instead of just saying, 'Look at me, I have a six pack.' The idea was always to do something completely left field and random; if it wasn't the pyjama company, I would've ventured into food seasonings or another food-based product. Excuse me, I'm talking as if I'm on my deathbed saying goodbye to what could've been. There is of course still time and I'll definitely be applying my marketing experience to a new business in the future.

In a nutshell, it's quite clear to see that millions can be made in the social media space. Whether you want to create a business from scratch or sell photos of your feet, the industry doesn't care and will pay you for your contribution (I cannot be certain of that actually, as I have not personally seen your feet). It's also fair for anyone outside of the industry to wonder if it's a viable source of income. You might not be ready to dive in head-first but, as I have recommended to a lot of the younger guys out there: build your platform, create a community and don't quit your day job until your side hustle can support you to go all in OR you're happy to bet on your willingness to make it happen and you need all the hours in a day that you physically have.

This doesn't have to be just about social media though. An underlying lesson that can be drawn from this is that, if you are in the top 5 per cent of your field, you can find a way to be rewarded for it. Just like I had no idea initially how to make money from my goal, I knew that if I succeeded in the field the money would follow. So whatever your vision is, don't be quick to dismiss it without fully understanding the bigger picture at hand.

*Reader closes book, inspired, and looks at chimp holding juggling balls.*

# 34
# A valuable lesson in selling your undies

After high school I went on to get my Bachelor of Commerce at the University of Melbourne. I graduated in 2018, majoring in finance and marketing. I studied principles of macroeconomics and learned the Keynesian theory. I studied microeconomics and learned all about the theory of markets and the elasticity of demand. But nothing taught me more about basic supply and demand than waking up to a direct message on my Instagram from a complete stranger, asking me if he could buy my undies.

Often I like to mess with people. When I get a message asking if my undies happen to be for sale as casually as you'd ask David Jones if their underwear is available to purchase, I am morally obliged to take the piss. You don't ask to buy David Jones's actual personal used and worn underwear, so I feel like I can have some fun.

I speak to a lot of other 'influencers' and they tell me the same thing regarding the so-called 'creeps' who make weird requests in their DMs: block them, delete them, 'They're weirdos mate, just block and move on.' A part of me knows that this is probably the right thing to do. But another part of me yearns to exploit the peculiarity for my own comedic gain.

So I proceeded to ask the young man a few questions, such as: Would he like worn undies or new ones? If they were extra sweaty would that incur additional costs? What colour would he prefer? Surprisingly, he answered them all as though they were genuine inquiries, like he'd done this before.

I was *this* close to walking into my dad's room, pinching some of his traumatised designer briefs and posting them straight to my new friend with an attached invoice, but I just couldn't do it. Why? Not for righteous reasons, that's for sure, but because he sent me a photo from my Instagram of me wearing a specific set of undies with the accompanying text, 'These ones.'

Great.

Thankfully I remembered some of my microeconomics. It was like a lightbulb went off in my undies. I remembered that the price you set is to maximise consumer's willingness to pay. We had established the product: used undies. Cool, now we just had to establish the price. Old mate could've gone down to his local shops and scored himself some brand-new undies for $20, yet he was more than willing to pay me $290 for my year-old, tattered and worn-out daks.

Imagine if I went down to the local shopping centre, found someone browsing through briefs and, with one hand down my pants, I interrupted him with an, 'Excuse me mate. I see you're interested in underwear. If you'd like these shitty old ones I'd be willing to settle for $300.' I'd either get hit or laughed at. But this guy right here was BEGGING for the sale, and I bet there are plenty of other lovely people like him who would do the same.

Fetishes aside, it actually demonstrates a valuable lesson in business that I use to this day: you don't need to sell to everyone, you just need to sell to the right customers and they will pay the right price. I applied this to my online coaching business and my pyjama business. When Joel and I launched our loungewear company, our costs were so high that we had no choice but to launch above the regular market price for pyjamas. We made in Australia using the best inputs we could find, hoping to be met with plenty of support. You get what you pay for right?

Well, we launched at 9am on 6 October 2021 and all we got was outrage from my Instagram followers. People were so disappointed at the price and they thought we were in the business of robbing people. We were called unfair and unethical. To us, knowing the quality of the product – not to mention that we both wore Slouch for over five hours per day, excluding sleeping – each pair was worth much more than our retail price. I remember sitting down at 9.05am in despair and saying to Joel that maybe no one is willing to pay that much for something you wear around the house. Pure sadness.

Then, by 9pm, we had sold nearly $70,000 worth of pyjamas. Happiness.

It occurred to us that we were 100 per cent right in saying that not everyone is willing to pay that high a price for pyjamas. In fact, if you surveyed everyone and found the average price that people would be willing to pay for pyjamas, or anything for that matter, it would be pitifully low. Probably a few cents. But we didn't need *everyone* to buy our product, we only needed a few hundred of the right people.

Bang. Another lightbulb in my undies moment.

# 35

# How to start a seven-figure business with zero experience

I called the fabric supplier to confirm their opening hours and, after an exciting two-hour drive, my brother and I stepped into their office. We were hoping this would be our answer: our way into the pyjama industry. I eagerly asked the lady I had spoken to on the phone what she had to show us. In my mind, she would present us with an array of recommended fabrics and instructions on making what we envisioned, with the next steps set up from there.

Instead of making our dream a reality, she crushed it almost immediately. She showed us to her office filled with tubs of hundreds of small pieces of fabric and said, unenthusiastically, 'Take a look.' Joel and I randomly felt pieces of fabric with completely unfamiliar names and compositions. Rayon with spandex, cotton with rayon, nylon with viscose, all different percentages. Panic set in as we realised we were in over our heads. After five minutes of arbitrarily feeling fabrics that all felt the same, we left feeling defeated. Mum called us as we were on our way home, expecting great news, and I was ready for Joel to tell her what a failure it had been and that the whole thing was a bad idea. Instead he just said, 'Yeah that one didn't really work out. She was an idiot. We're going to stop at every fabric supplier on our way home.'

That optimism set the tone for the next three years.

We stopped at the closest fabric supplier we could locate on Google and walked into a huge warehouse. We approached a man on a forklift and Joel immediately started telling him about us and our plan to make pyjamas in Melbourne. He basically told this guy our entire vision for the company, Slouch Potato.

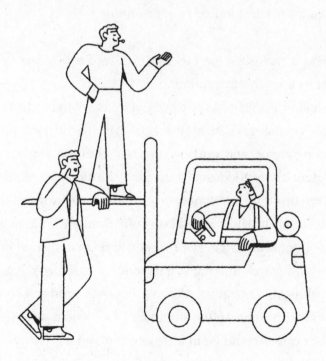

The man on the forklift didn't speak a word of English, but he kindly directed us to the front office. The ladies in there were a little more helpful and gave us their opinion on what would make a nice fabric for pyjamas. The most helpful thing they said was that we would need to find a manufacturer to make them. Our naive minds had thought that a supplier and a manufacturer were one and the same. Just add that to the expanding list of things we didn't know but were willing to learn.

It felt good to get back to the drawing board. We checked out Alibaba to try and find our dream manufacturer. We sent companies a Microsoft Paint-style mock-up of pyjama pants, annotated with crude measurements of things that don't even need to be measured, and surprisingly they sent back a product. It was probably the worst thing I've ever seen in my life.

So we canned Alibaba and continued our search for a manufacturer and supplier closer to home.

This was a new deal for Joel and me, and a business venture both of us knew nothing about.

Growing up we always wore pyjamas. We may have been the only young guys in high school who would look forward to coming home and putting on their comfiest clothes. We'd completely understood and harnessed the elements of self-care achieved through developing a consistent evening routine of getting out of the shower and into your comfiest, softest clothes. The routine would trigger our minds to relax and wind down.

So the idea of making a garment we loved *even better* was extraordinarily appealing. We saw how the products could be improved (through a softer, stretchier fabric and a better fit) and how the designs could be made more fun and less corny.

Before this venture I had been wary about the idea of starting a clothing company, because the business seemed way over my head and I felt like I had as much of an eye for design as an underground mole. But this felt different for some reason. Maybe it was because I was doing something with my best friend (my brother) and we had a vision for what we wanted to create.

The roadblock of being completely uninformed still remained, however. So we set out on a mission to start from scratch and learn the process. We researched how a clothing company is made. What a fabric supplier was, what a manufacturer did, how to create patterns for clothing fits and the various methods of printing fabrics. Unlike the first lady we spoke to, whom I shall refer to eloquently as 'the idiot', our next fabric supplier was exactly what we needed. His name is Stephen and his advice has been invaluable. We weren't afraid to ask questions and he was happy to answer them.

Stephen gave us a list of manufacturers and we called them that day. Most declined, believing that we would be just another start-up wasting their time, but we continued until we found someone to make them for us. We finally had a product and Slouch Potato was born.

Joel and I designed the prints for the pants. We found a talented graphic designer to bring them to life and then together figured out how to make it a repeatable pattern. We travelled across Australia to visit a fabric-printing company, sent them almost a kilometre of our fabric and, after months of trial and error, they came back with a successfully printed test (strike off) for us to approve.

Then we were slapped with the invoice: $60 printing per metre. That would mean $60,000 just to print our fabric, bringing our cost to make pyjamas to well over $150 per pair. The business model didn't work so back to the drawing board we went, until we finally had a viable model and a working sample.

I wish I could say that our mistakes ended there.

Our first range came back entirely different to what we'd described. There must've been confusion in our sampling process (or lack thereof) because our T-shirts had sleeves far shorter than we intended and our loose-fitting pant legs were now tight. Oh well, at least we had a product that was usable, after 18 months of work. I marketed it as best as I could to my social media following, and on the day of launching we exceeded our expectations.

As I said, some people were outraged by the price. After 18 months of work and well over six figures of my own personal investment, I had to explain myself and our pricing to people online. We ignored any pointless negativity, took whatever constructive criticism we could and never stopped learning.

Joel quit his job as a house framer and we gave this new company everything we had. He learned the specifics about manufacturing garments and how to utilise people's skill sets. He was relentless when it came down to it. I marketed our vision and deliberated with Joel every day on the smallest of decisions. We were pushing against what seemed like a closed door, as not many of my gym-loving followers had bought pyjamas in their life, yet we were trying to communicate the value to them.

Thankfully, our vision seemed to resonate. When asked about the value of our product, it wasn't just our opinion: it was factual. No one could tell me they didn't like being comfortable at home and no one could tell me they had a more comfortable alternative than what we made. Putting two and two together we could tell people, this is what you wear any time you're at home for maximum comfort. The sales didn't come easy and we had to grind for the rest of the year to both continue developing and making our product better and more efficient, all while communicating to the world why they needed it.

Luckily the people that did buy Slouch became repeat customers. After a year of business, we had sold nearly half a million dollars' worth of pyjamas.

We must've been stoked right? Two young guys making five hundred grand in their first year of business. Well, every dollar earned went back into the business to pay everyone involved. There wasn't even a single dollar left for us to split between us. If this was a get-rich-quick scheme, it definitely did not work. But we were stoked.

We had learned how to create a product from nothing. We had entered an entirely new industry and created a clothing brand, despite having zero experience. All we had was a desire to learn and a vision, and I credit all we achieved to that. The vision is what kept us going and the desire to learn was what would get us there. The same attitude that caused us to accept our first defeat enabled us to continue taking beatings in the hope that something good will come. We wanted every household and young person wearing our products. We knew the immense value they would provide because they had done so for us personally.

I think it's cool that two brothers with just an idea can turn it into something real that adds value to thousands of people all over the world. I'm not telling you this to flex or to proclaim that we've 'made it', but more to share the underlying lesson.

We knew absolutely nothing about the clothing industry. But we *learned*, and it's as simple as that.

I get a lot of people asking me what they should do, because they do not possess a particular set of skills. After clarifying that they're not Liam Neeson, I tell them that it doesn't matter. If we can learn this much from nothing, so can you. You just need to be able to take things one step at a time, be patient, ask experts to share their knowledge and be willing to learn everything you can about your chosen venture. It doesn't have to be much more complicated than that.

Many people struggle with this concept and do not move past it. Typically, people will start out then realise that they don't possess the desired skill to do x, y or z, and then get angry about their lack of possibility and potential as if they are stuck forever. Some of the best advice I ever received was to figure out the specific skills you need to make money, assess your own skill set and identify those you do not yet have, and then go out and learn them to bridge the gap.

The idea that you can learn anything with time is unbelievably empowering. Don't see your inadequacies as limitations; see them as areas to direct your focus to or simply as things you haven't mastered *yet*. And finally, if you are starting something and you feel embarrassed about your lack of knowledge, just remember Joel pitching his heart out to a man on a forklift in Melbourne's industrial area, with nothing but an idea.

# 36

# The unexpected gift of social media

Miami, 15 May 2022. I step out of the shower, wrap the towel around myself and attempt to dry my body in record time. My back is still wet but I throw a T-shirt on anyway. Call it a flexibility issue or just pure laziness, but this is quite normal for me. I walk out of my bedroom and into the open living room, admire the view from the 30th floor and see my videographer Hafiy waiting for me, camera in hand. We head downstairs to meet the taxi. Despite it being a near two-hour trip to see my friend, I'm excited. The taxi smells like cigarettes and 10 expired air fresheners, but the driver is happy to get a $150 trip and bombs it down the highway at 150km per hour … while on her phone … typing AND talking.

Obviously I don't die. We arrive in one piece and knock three times on my mate's door. A large figure approaches on the other side and welcomes us in with a big grin. 'Hey man! It's been a long time,' says Chris, as he goes for a bro hug and makes me feel like a scrawny child hugging his dad.

I first met Chris Bumstead (also known as CBum) at a Gymshark event in Toronto, Canada. This was before he was crowned Mr Olympia and became a mega successful businessman, but he still has the same humble, down-to-earth attitude today as he had then. We immediately hit it off and became mates. This happens quite easily when two people have very similar interests and are in similar positions. We both had a passion for bodybuilding (he was just a thousand times better than me at it) and we both had aspirations for succeeding in our own ways.

Many of my closest friends today live on the other side of the world. In fact, as I worked on this book, I was in Thailand on a trip with two other couples that I first met online and have become great friends with. I've been to Ibiza, Bali, Japan, London, Kenya, Dubai and the United States, all with new friends I made on social media. It sounds crazy to develop friendships this way, but that's one true positive that social media offers: human connection. Funnily enough, that's the entire point behind it all, before it developed its money-hungry evil persona that wants to steal your attention and sell it to the highest bidder.

Social media gets a lot of flack for the many real downsides to it (some of which we will go into in the next chapter) but it has an immense power to connect like-minded people, unbound by geography or time zones.

Even during my early days on social media as an up-and-coming fitness creator, I connected with many of the same kind of people and we constantly rooted for each other's success. This was a breath of fresh air and one of many contributing factors to my success today. The people I'd usually surround myself with in 'real life' were supportive in one sense but also would take friendly digs (as most mates would do), which would cause me to doubt myself.

I simply could not have any doubt in my mind or in my circle when trying to achieve something bigger than myself. I needed to create an environment of positivity and shared vision so that when it got hard, I had the right people to lean on and ask for help.

If you're on a fat-loss journey, it helps to join groups online where people can post their progress judgement free and get genuine help and feedback. I invite all of my coaching clients to my private group on Facebook for this reason. Thousands of people were shocked at how they could post photos of themselves that they could *never* allow to be seen on their own profiles, yet they'd be met with encouragement and praise when they posted them in my group.

Why were these people terrified to post on their own profile? Because they were posting full-blown nudes, with their wiener in a death grip and wearing a huge grin. I'm kidding, obviously they were worried their own friends and family would judge them, ridicule them or doubt them for posting a simple fitness photo. Sometimes it's easier to trust strangers than your own friends and family – that is a clear enough reason to expand your social circle.

Social media is a great way for us to craft our own social environment and experience a sense of belonging that we all long to have. During the pandemic, people had no choice but to use social media for its original purpose and connect with loved ones and create new friendships (let's just pretend that the loonies didn't capitalise on this a little too much). We had Zoom calls with friends, fostered new passions and bonded over shared interests.

If it wasn't for social media, I wouldn't feel the same level of connection with people all over the world. For me especially, the feeling of contribution and connection I have to hundreds of thousands of people world-wide is mind boggling. When people watch my videos, they feel like they know me. When they meet me in person, they have in-jokes already at their disposal and I can tell that's weird for them because *they believe* that we're friends and at the same time we both know full well that I don't know who the hell they are. The amount of times someone's told me this is hilarious.

To think that I can have a positive effect on someone and can create meaningful connection is the life force of my actions. That feeling is what keeps me filming videos and posting content, even when it all goes south. For example, in the past I've gone through phases where YouTube decided to completely shit on my channel (as far as reach goes). I could barely monetise and couldn't even justify the costs of production. Despite these feelings of negativity and hopelessness, I'd continue to film and edit week after week, because I knew that somewhere out there someone could benefit from my video. That one thing I say could potentially be the one thing to change someone's life.

That level of contribution and connection cannot be matched by money or anything tangible. It's the driving purpose that fuels my everyday actions and it's the reason why I'm writing this book.

If you use it wisely and correctly, social media can be a warm and welcoming environment that can push you to that next level. It can be a vessel of genuine connection, information dissemination and love transportation. However, if used incorrectly or absentmindedly, it can be destructive, toxic and severely damaging to one's mental health. Sadly, 'it ain't all sunshine and rainbows.'

# 37

# The intimate downsides of social media

An introduction to a stranger is usually followed by the question, 'What do you do?' In the event that I answer truthfully (and don't give them a vague answer such as 'I work in fitness' to avoid any further questions), a lot of guys follow this up by asking in a blokey-bloke manner, 'Wow, you must do all right with the ladies, eh?' Wink wink, nudge nudge and whatever other clichéd, supposedly masculine gesture fits the scene.

As painful as it is, I always give them a beautifully ambiguous, 'I've done okay!' to cease conversation on the topic. The truth is, I probably didn't do okay. In my opinion, if someone has attention of any kind, be it on social media or through traditional media, it can have a dramatic effect on their relationships with others, and especially with dating. One obvious effect is that the person could take advantage of their position of power or influence and sleep with as many people as possible, wading through a sea of initials (STD, NDA ...) in the process, until they come to a realisation that something has to change. A less obvious path is one of paranoia and insecurity, and leads to withdrawing into oneself and refusing to trust anyone else.

The latter is what I experienced as I started to develop a public name for myself. Thankfully I no longer feel the same way as I did in my early 20s, but at the time I created quite a lonely and isolated existence for myself. I had experienced people attempt to use me for my 'clout' (horrible word but it does a great job at describing the intangible, meaningless weight of one's popularity), which caused me to retreat even more into my shell. This was the first true downside of social media that I experienced personally. Here's what happened ...

This all started when guys my age would spend every day swiping dating apps until they'd show early signs of repetitive strain injuries in their thumb. They'd be talking to girls, catching up with girls and mainly focusing on girls. For me, I had an enormous goal hanging over my head. I didn't really let myself think about girls and I sought comfort in my ability to not need anyone else, because all I needed to achieve my goal was myself, without distractions.

My ambition became my only focus and sadly I became used to being alone. For a while I stopped actively seeking out girls altogether because I was so deep in my routine of work, gym and content creation in order to facilitate my goal. I once took a girl out on a date because I thought that's what I should have been doing. I did it not because I wanted to spend time with her, but because I felt the need to conform to societal expectation.

In addition to this, I also had problems with ego and trust.

While guys were swiping maniacally, I was being *sent* dating-app profiles of me that I hadn't created. One guy was called Chad and he was a 26-year-old model. Another Zac was named Robert and he was actually a doctor! I'm still upset to this day that someone thought I looked like a Chad. Girls would send me these catfishes to either flatter me or let me know in case I wanted to do anything about it. However, the only thing it made me want to do was not be on any dating app. I felt like it would be embarrassing if I tried to engage in conversation only for a girl to screenshot my actual profile then send that to my actual Instagram for cross-referencing validation. I envisioned replying back to the hypothetical girl on Instagram, awkwardly saying, 'Hello. Yes it's me. Can you please reply to my message on Tinder?'

In hindsight it was an ego problem. Who even cares if I had to send that message? But back then it seemed embarrassing and I immediately placed myself *above* that, so I didn't use dating apps.

My trust issues began out of not knowing people's true intentions. I had girls that never looked at me all of a sudden think I was really nice and funny once I had millions of eyes on me. I couldn't tell whether a girl actually wanted to date me for me or if they were influenced by my so-called influence. That idea contributed to my existing insecurities, so the easiest way for me to deal with it at the time was to avoid it altogether.

Instead of dating girls who didn't know who I was, or finding ones who weren't swayed by social media, I had a false picture in my head of what they might be thinking. It was an immature and limiting assumption that gave me an even bigger excuse to not let anyone in and to be even more alone. On the occasion that I would go on a date, any potential red flags would confirm my assumptions that they didn't actually care about me.

I was at a restaurant once, taking photos of my delicious food, when the girl asked me to tag her in the post – knowing full well that she was not the subject depicted in the photo and isn't in fact a shallow-fried squid. Now, I know that clearly this is more of a reflection on the type of person I was choosing to surround myself with and less of a representation of the actual situation at hand, but everything is clearer in retrospect. At the time I couldn't see past my blinding distrust.

I would be very hesitant to make new friends. To some degree I still am today, yet through experience I have developed quite a good gauge on who is genuine and who wants something. I play it safe and only let a few people truly in. I have friends, I don't *need* more, but if it happens I'm open to it.

Now back to dating. I haven't described when this loneliness stopped or if it even did.

I became so accustomed to being lonely, it didn't really feel like loneliness anymore. It just felt like the way things were. Particularly in my case, when I had hundreds of strangers – guys and girls alike – praising me online while I was keeping my life completely to myself. I didn't let anyone in and didn't seek anyone else. I was literally creating my own isolation out of a fear of being judged, embarrassed, used or hurting my own ego.

I was 23 years old when I found the first girl I even thought about having a relationship with. Her personality was refreshing and I didn't have to try to make anything work. Except for the fact that she lived in another country; after a couple of trips back and forth it didn't work out. However, that brief phase reminded me how good it can be to experience things with someone else.

Common sense, right? You're probably nodding your head thinking, 'Yeah, no shit, who wants to be alone?' But before that,

I hadn't even questioned myself. But I started to deal with my anxieties around dating. It took a lot of thinking, real-world experience and meeting the right people. I stopped looking for girls who might want everything I was afraid they'd want: fame, attention, superficial association or clout. I tried to look for the right person for me. For me, looking for the right person was harder than settling for someone, but it was worth it. This shift contributed to a huge growth in my own character.

I wasn't going to include this chapter in in this book, as I wasn't too sure who would even want to hear about my unimpressive failed relationships or a dry streak that would impress the Sahara Desert, but I think it's worth mentioning that looks may be deceiving. I'm not a grotesque-looking person and usually any kind of fame would imply a smooth run with the ladies, but my experience was far from that. For a time in my life I sought to be alone. One the other hand, the last thing I would want is a dependence on someone else for my own happiness. However, just like anything else in life, there needs to be a balance. Despite my willingness to be alone, I also needed to grow as a person and be willing to let people in. Since then, I've found relationships that have made me a much happier person than I was by myself. I'm a better person for it. But to get to where I am now I had to stop overthinking, cease being consumed by irrational fears, trust people, put my ego aside and be less selfish.

Now I sleep with more women than I ever dreamed of and have a new one for every day of the week. And you can too if you just sign up to my course at just $899.

Hopefully we're close enough now for you to know when I'm joking.

# 38

# Comparison: control it before it controls you

Theodore Roosevelt, Mark Twain and the Bible have all quoted variations of the idea that comparison is the thief of joy. It wasn't until my experience with social media that I truly came to understand the truth behind this message and the danger that lies in the act of comparison.

If I think back to the days before social media, my opportunities to compare myself were minuscule. I could only compare myself to the people around me, who turned out to be my brother and my friends.

James was a classic example. I met James when I was four years old and we soon became best friends, which we were throughout primary school. He was one of those kids that was just a natural at sports. Every year he'd get the MVP award in our basketball team. I'd be there with my fingers crossed, hoping that by some miracle the coaches would see my hidden talent lying dormant and say, 'You know what, I've had a change of heart. This year's MVP goes to Zac Perna for displaying heart and courage during his time on the bench.'

I wasn't particularly great at sport and would often look to James as my own point of reference for the best of the best and as inspiration. I wished I had his talent but, like my height, some things just had to be accepted. I was left unaffected for the most part. Then came high school.

I took it as a personal challenge to try to get top marks from day one. School projects became hobbies, homework became practice and any test or exam was merely a chance for me to show up to game day and try for the academic MVP. James, on the other hand, would sit there on the day of Year 7 exams, doubt his abilities and work himself up into a storm of anxiety, knowing he'd surely fail. In the weeks prior to the test, I'd console him, gas him up and tell him that we'd figure it out together.

Results day came around and he didn't fail ... but he felt like he had. He received a B+. Compared to failing, a B+ is a mark to make anyone ecstatic. But James would look at my consistent stream of As and A+s, then look at his marks and *feel* like a failure. This went on for quite some time. James was in fact a very bright kid, and averaging 75 per cent is great by anyone's standards, but that's the way it goes when your standard is set to that of those around you.

The problem with social media is that it expands the number of people you can set your standard against to an unfathomably large amount. If you want to, you can connect to billions of people. You can find millions of people who are more skilled than you are at your hobby, your job and your interests. The number of people connected in an instant is truly unfathomable in the most literal sense: the human mind can only hold and process a certain number of connections. The Dunbar rule says that that number is 150. Beyond that, it's theorised that we lose our ability to function effectively in social relationships. It makes sense, evolutionarily speaking. Tribes are small. Our brains have carefully adapted to this fact. Then we put a smartphone with a few apps in front of our face and all of a sudden we are holding a gateway to a perceivably infinite number of connections.

I experienced this when I was already making a living from social media. The people I'd follow on Instagram would be other fitness creators and fitness models, and there was no shortage of physiques better than mine. As a result, my confidence in my body plummeted through the floor. Every day I'd see 50 physiques far better than mine. And because fitness was my focus, Instagram was definitely not showing me the average body on the street, but rather more of what it thought I'd be interested in.

So I'd continue scrolling and scrolling past the genetic freaks, shredded strangers and jacked giants until I put my phone down and came back to the real world with a sense that something was lost. My intuition was right. I had literally lost happiness and self-worth after comparing myself to people at a completely surface level. I didn't ask these people how their relationships with their family were, what their happiness looked like or anything else that might paint a holistic picture of them as a person. I just looked at their appearance and created the narrative that they were simply better than me. Boom! Another decrease in happiness. The cycle continued and this became my reality – what you focus on becomes what you experience.

In hindsight, I can see that this upward comparison never ends, but at the time I was too entrenched in the moment. I felt like I just had to be better all of the time. After many months, I realised that something had to change because, at the rate I was going, I was never going to catch the goal because the goal was constantly moving.

I remember checking my phone in the morning and wondering why I felt slightly worse after just a few minutes of scrolling (this is why I removed my phone from my morning routine, which you will remember from chapter 8). I can now see why. If it wasn't the physical body it was something else. Someone always seemed to have a better life than me. At some point I realised that *I* was that person to someone else. Aha! The infinite loop of negative comparison was revealed.

People are biologically programmed to compare upwards, never downwards. Upward comparison forces action and drives growth. We choose what success looks like in our eyes and we upwardly compare in a dopamine-seeking pursuit. In the past perhaps this wasn't too bad because, as I experienced with James, you'd win some and you'd lose some. I never got the MVP in basketball but I definitely improved in skills, and I was happy with that. James never got perfect marks every time, but he definitely had his fair share of As.

I'd rather surround myself with people better than me at certain skills or more successful than me in certain fields for this exact reason. And this is manageable when the size of your circle of comparison is limited to a few people or even Dunbar's 150 at the very most. But when it's only limited by the estimated half of the world's population who are online (4.26 billion people), it feels infinitely large and dredges up feelings of worthlessness, anxiety and hopelessness.

We have to catch ourselves in periods of online comparison and stop it in its tracks.

So how do we fix this? How did I fix this? With gratitude and perspective.

You cannot be truly grateful and be in a state of dissatisfied 'wanting' at the same time. Gratitude displaces feelings of comparison or low self-worth. True gratitude fills your cup and comparison drains it, but thankfully you can only focus intently on one at a time. For me, realising this helped immensely. Every time I'd catch myself in a negative loop of comparing, I'd think about everything that I had. I'd think that someone out there would kill to have my life. I'd count my blessings in the most literal sense and try to really feel the gratitude.

I don't just look in the mirror and say to myself, 'I'm grateful for my family and friends,' while wondering if affirmations even work or why I sound like an idiot. I imagine what it would be like to have them all stripped from me. I imagine someone out there experiencing that dread in reality. I do this at a visceral level because it's the only way I can develop a true understanding for what it is that I have. At this level, the comparison points are trivial and are drowned out by present gratitude for what I have. For a while, I feel rich.

I think everyone needs to pair any form of comparison with a sense of perspective and gratitude that can refill the joy that has been depleted. Without gratitude and perspective, people will continue down this never-ending loop of negativity until there is no joy left. That's the ending because the prize never comes. The end result will always be ever so slightly out of reach and you'll rob yourself of happiness before you ever get there.

So that's what I do. I avoid any comparisons on social media because I know it's extremely biased. I also avoid comparing my success to my own past successes. Because even the act of doing that is placing your mind in a negative loop of thinking that keeps you living in the past and not grateful for the present.

I only compare myself as a person using intangibles. I compare my values over time because those are truly influenced and controlled by me. Success comes and goes and winning is a non-linear path. But if I can look back and say to myself that I've grown as a person, that I'm living more in line with my own values, that I'm passing along the lessons that I've learned to those who need it, then I can successfully harness the action of comparison for good.

# Conclusion

You know that point in a conversation where you and your companion both know it's coming to an end, so you start reeling off the classic conversation enders in a downward inflection like 'aaaanyway', 'oh well ...' or 'that was fun' only to walk away in the same direction and awkwardly laugh it off, having to have yet another concluding conversation? No? Never happened to you? Oh well. Aaaanyway, that was fun and I hope you also enjoyed our conversation. I'll see you later. You're still reading? The book is done now. You can stop reading. This is awkward.

Well, if you are still reading then I have to admit that I am excited for you. You have all of the tools at your disposal to live your best life. Whether your goal is to get into your best shape, burn fat, build muscle, feel great, start a business or crush social media, you have the choice to do it all. You can command a greater power over your mind, improve your mental health and decide that you want to see what YOU are fully capable of. You've heard from me and hopefully can take one or two lessons out of my fun and sometimes messy journey and apply them to your own life right now. Because you deserve to feel great in your own mind and body. You deserve to be boldly ambitious and demand more from your life. So don't let any motivation be fleeting and useless. Turn it into action right now and start living the life that you deserve.

Ever since I was 10 years old I had dreams of helping people – of being a doctor; a surgeon actually. I knew it was a respected career and ultimately I wanted to help other people and make a difference. My grades were good and I wasn't squeamish, so the career path seemed like the perfect fit. Then when I was 12 I slammed my finger in the garage door so hard that the paramedics couldn't decipher which bits were bone and which were nail. While they learned the difference, I learned what the word 'squeamish' meant. I resisted the urge to faint and vomit while ruling out my chosen career path.

After that, I didn't know what I wanted to do with my life. All I knew was that one day I was going to make a difference in people's lives and that was one dream that no one could rule out for me. I never imagined that *this* would be my way of making a difference. I continue to do what I do and strive to be better. There are people out there that need help in some way or another, and I wrote this book for those people. I decided to fill these pages and create somewhat of a handbook because the road that I took to get here was not a smooth one. It was rocky, full of potholes and had enough corners and bends to force me to pull over and throw up, wondering how I possibly could even finish the journey. But it doesn't have to be that way for everyone. You can take both the straight road and the shortcut.

I made the many mistakes I did because I had no other option. In fact, I think I made every mistake humanly possible. The alternative title of this book could've been *Bad Shit: The dumb things that I did so that you don't have to*. I stumbled and fumbled my way to a better life because I had to. I had no choice but to just try and move forward, even if that meant years of moving backwards at times. I spent 14 years focusing on how to master the physical body, how to create a mindset to allow sustainable change and unlimited potential and how to create a career out of my passions. My goal is to save you from the bad advice I was given, the unnecessarily hard path, and instead provide a means to learn from my mistakes and still achieve a life-changing result on your own.

I didn't write this book with the intention of it being loved by all or praised by everyone. I wrote this book with the goal of becoming a good influence on just one person. I hope that one particular nugget of information may be the catalyst that drives at least one person's life in a better direction. It goes without saying that I don't have all of the answers. I still need Google Maps to direct me back to my house outside of a 5km radius, and I still make my bed like an escaped psychopath. But I have managed to improve thousands of physiques and, most importantly, changed my own life along the way.

As you probably understand by now, no one is going to do this for you. No one can. It is now up to you to compile worthwhile takeaways from these pages and get to work. Hopefully you have found some helpful advice and can go back, highlight the most applicable content and study it, turning it into action items that you can do right now to live a life just fractionally better tomorrow. Even if it is just the act of going for a walk with a loved one, having a laugh with a good friend or dressing up as Harry Potter. Although maybe avoid giving Nando's wraps to buskers. That would be embarrassing.

I definitely do not have all of the answers, but I hope that these confessions can help you in some way, or at the very least, just entertain you as I invite you into the inner workings of the weird and wonderful world of my life as a social media 'influencer'. It truly pains me to write that word, but in the word's defence, my dreams have always been to influence others to lead a better life. Even if I'm still finding my own feet and don't have everything figured out, at the heart and soul of it, my only dream in life is to be a good influence. Consider this my formal attempt.

Much Love, Zac.

# Acknowledgements

I have a lot of people to thank for this book considering it is an amalgamation of over a decade of learning, struggling, failing and succeeding. It would be impossible to name every person that has contributed – my friends know who they are.

I'll begin by thanking my family, the people I've mentioned most throughout this book, for their impact on both my life and the writing of *Good Influence*. I am fortunate to have a family that has supported me – from my first goal to join the gym to the milestone of publishing a book. To my mum, Trina, thanks for always being my number one fan in whatever I do and for the positivity and optimism that any son would be so lucky to have. Also, thanks for correcting my grammar in the random pieces of writing that I did – who knows what kind of writer I would've been without an avid reader for a mother? To my dad, Sam, for being a brilliant role model for me and my first 'good influence'. Thank you for bouncing ideas back and forth and for your constant encouragement. To my brother, Joel: supporter, training partner, business partner and, most importantly, lifetime best friend. Thank you for starting me off on my fitness journey and inspiring me to aim high and imagine the best possible outcome in every opportunity life has thrown.

To the incredible team at HarperCollins Publishers, I have no idea where to start because without you all this would still be a dream of mine. I have many people to thank both indirectly and directly. To Mary Rennie, my incredible publisher, thank you for putting your faith in me and bringing me into the publishing scene. Your insights and curiosity are world-class. To the outstanding editorial team for making this book the best it could possibly be. And to the rest of publishing powerhouse HarperCollins for being so welcoming and accommodating and acting as my very own support network.

A big thanks to Joseph Carrington of Moses Illustration for bringing my wild ideas to life on the page in your awesome and unique illustration style.

Last of all, my final thank you is to YOU reading this: for supporting me and always choosing a better life for yourself. Never stop levelling up, because you are incredible and deserve the very best that life can offer.

# Endnotes

**5. Get bloody cold**

1   Wim Hof, *The Wim Hof Method*, Sounds True, United States, 2020.
2   P Šrámek, M Šimečková, L Janský, et al, 'Human physiological responses to immersion into water of different temperatures' *Eur J Appl Physiol*, March 2000; https://pubmed.ncbi.nlm.nih.gov/10751106/

**12. The body's superpower**

3   AV Nedeltcheva, JM Kilkus, J Imperial, DA Schoeller, PD Penev, 'Insufficient sleep undermines dietary efforts to reduce adiposity', *Ann Intern Med*, October 2010; https://pubmed.ncbi.nlm.nih.gov/20921542/
4   Matthew Walker, *Why We Sleep*, Scribner, United Kingdom, 2018
5   Dr Sachin Panda, *The Circadian Code*, Random House, United Kingdom, 2018

**15. My very own origin story**

6   Australian Bureau of Statistics, 'National Health Survey: First results', 12 December 2018; https://www.abs.gov.au/statistics/health/health-conditions-and-risks/national-health-survey-first-results/latest-release#health-risk-factors

**17. My own personal recipe for fat loss made easy**

7   JM Frecka, RD Mattes, 'Possible entrainment of ghrelin to habitual meal patterns in humans', *Am J Physiol Gastrointest Liver Physiol*, March 2008; https://pubmed.ncbi.nlm.nih.gov/18187517/

8   Y Wang, R Chandra, LA Samsa, B Gooch, BE Fee, JM Cook, SR
    Vigna, AO Grant, RA Liddle, 'Amino acids stimulate cholecystokinin
    release through the Ca2+-sensing receptor', *Am J Physiol Gastrointest
    Liver Physiol*, April 2011; https://pubmed.ncbi.nlm.nih.gov/21183662/
9   C Saner, AM Senior, H Zhang, AM Eloranta, CG Magnussen, MA
    Sabin, J Juonala, M Janner, DP Burgner, U Schwab, EA Haapala,
    BL Heitmann, SJ Simpson, D Raubenheimer, TA Lakka, 'Evidence
    for Protein Leverage in Children and Adolescents with Obesity',
    *Obesity (Silver Spring)*, April 2020; https://pubmed.ncbi.nlm.nih.
    gov/32144892/
10  KD Hall, A Ayuketa, R Brychta, H Cai, T Cassimatis, KY Chen,
    ST Chung, E Costa, A Courville, V Darcey, LA Fletcher, CG Forde,
    AM Gharib, J Gio, R Howard, PV Joseph, S McGehee, R Ouwekerk,
    K Raisinger, I Rozga, M Stagliano, M Walter, PJ Walter, S Yang,
    M Zhou, 'Ultra- Processed Diets Cause Excess Calorie Intake and
    Weight Gain: An Inpatient Randomized Controlled Trial of Ad
    Libitum Food Intake', *Cell Metab*, July 2019; https://pubmed.ncbi.nlm.
    nih.gov/31105044/

**20. The answer to stubborn fat**
11  BI Campbell, D Aguilar, LM Colenso-Semple, K Hartke, AR
    Fleming, CD Fox, JM Longstrom, GE Rogers, DB Mathas, V Wong,
    S Ford, J Gorman, 'Intermittent Energy Restriction Attenuates
    the Loss of Fat Free Mass in Resistance Trained Individuals. A
    Randomized Controlled Trial', *J Funct Morphol Kinesiol*, March 2020;
    https://pubmed.ncbi.nlm.nih.gov/33467235/

**22. Thou shalt not out-traineth a diet lacking valour**
12  Aishwarya Kumar, 'The grandmaster diet: How to lose weight while
    barely moving', *ESPN*, 27 April 2020; https://www.espn.com.au/
    espn/story/_/id/27593253/why-grandmasters-magnus-carlsen-
    fabiano-caruana-lose-weight-playing-chess

**24. How to create the perfect fat loss diet in five minutes**
13  JD Cameron, MJ Cyr, E Doucet, 'Increased meal frequency does not
    promote greater weight loss in subjects who were prescribed an 8-week
    equi-energetic energy-restricted diet', *Br J Nutr*, April 2010; https://
    pubmed.ncbi.nlm.nih.gov/19943985/

**25. Train for life, build muscle and avoid injuries**
14  D Plotkin, M Coleman, D Van Every, J Maldonado, D Oberlin, M
    Israetel, J Feather, A Alto, AD Vigotsky, BJ Schoenfeld, 'Progressive
    overload without progressing load? The effects of load or repetition

progression on muscular adaptations', *PeerJ*, 30 September 2022; https://pubmed.ncbi.nlm.nih.gov/36199287/

15   Chris Beardsley, 'What determines mechanical tension during strength training?', *Medium*, 15 November 2018; https://sandcresearch.medium.com/what-determines-mechanical-tension-during-strength-training-acdf31b93e18#:~:text=In%20fact%2C%20contraction%20velocity%20determines,to%20the%20force%2Dvelocity%20relationship

16   Martin Refalo, & Eric Helms, & David Hamilton, & Jackson Fyfe, 'Towards an improved understanding of proximity-to-failure in resistance training and its influence on skeletal muscle hypertrophy, neuromuscular fatigue, muscle damage, and perceived discomfort: A scoping review', *Journal of Sports Sciences*, June 2022; https://pubmed.ncbi.nlm.nih.gov/35658845/

## 27. Small changes for HUGE results

17   Astrup Arne, 'The satiating power of protein—a key to obesity prevention?', *The American Journal of Clinical Nutrition*, July 2005; https://pubmed.ncbi.nlm.nih.gov/16002791/

18   JW Apolzan, CA Myers, CM Champagne, RA Beyl, HA Raynor, SA Anton, S.A., DA Williamson, FM Sacks, GA Bray, and CK Martin, 'Frequency of Consuming Foods Predicts Changes in Cravings for Those Foods During Weight Loss: The POUNDS Lost Study', *Obesity (Silver Spring)*, August 2017; https://www.ncbi.nlm.nih.gov/pmc/articles/PMC5529244/#:~:text=Altering%20frequency%20of%20consuming%20craved,not%20appear%20to%20alter%20cravings.